Prep Your Way
Workshops | Online Courses | Workbooks

Associate Safety Professional (ASP)

Certified Instructional Trainer (CIT)

Certified Hazardous Materials Manager (CHMM)

Construction Health and Safety Technician (CHST)

Certified Industrial Hygienist (CIH)

Certified Safety Professional (CSP)

Occupational Hygiene and Safety Technologist (OHST)

Safety Management Specialist (SMS)

Safety Trained Supervisor (STS)

Safety Trained Supervisor Construction (STSC)

SPAN™ **Exam Prep** is the leading certification exam study solution to prepare safety professionals for exams from the Board of Certified Safety Professionals (BCSP). This BCSP exam prep helps professionals achieve important career goals through advancing competencies for safety management excellence. As the leader in BCSP exam preparation since 1992, SPAN offers live workshops, online courses and workbooks. The self-directed study materials are designed for professionals looking to gain critical knowledge, study techniques, and testing strategies to pass certification examinations.

www.spansafety.com

Dedicated to All Safety, Health and Environmental Professionals

Striving to Protect

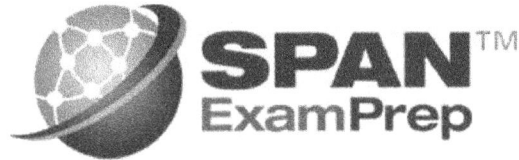

SPAN™
ExamPrep

www.spansafety.com

This Publication is not intended to guarantee that the user will pass an exam, become certified or in general may not cover every aspect of the certification process.

The information contained in this study workbook is intended to be used in preparation for the Occupational Hygiene and Safety Technician® examination and should not be used as an authority in the professional practice of safety, health, or environmental compliance.

The Occupational Hygiene and Safety Technician® (OHST®) Certification is a registered trademark of the Board of Certified Safety Professionals (BCSP). The opinions expressed are those of the authors and no guarantee, warranty, or other representation is made as to the absolute correctness or sufficiency of any information contained in this study workbook.

Daniel J. Snyder, Ed.D, CSP, OHST
Copyright © 2019 by SPAN™ International Training, LLC
402 W. Mt Vernon St #111
Nixa, Missouri 65714
Phone: 417 724 8348
info@spansafetyworkshops.com

ISBN 978-1-886786-28-8 (set)
ISBN 978-1-886786-26-4 (v.1)
ISBN 978-1-886786-27-1 (v.2)

Table of Contents

Self-Assessment Practice Exams

This section of the workbook provides a practice examination that has one hundred questions and answers like those on the OHST examination. The average time per question on the exam is about one minute. Complete teach 100 questions self-assessment exam in 90 minutes.

Self-Assessment Exam One Questions

1) The term anhydrous in *anhydrous ammonia* means:

    A) 100% pure.
    B) Without water.
    C) Without impurities.
    D) Hospital Grade.

2) Determine the pH of a solution in which [H+] = 2.3 x 10^{-5} Moles per liter.

    A) -4.64 mild acid.
    B) 4.64 mild acid.
    C) 12.3 strong base.
    D) -12.3 strong base.

3) A lead weight weighs 1400 ounces on land. It weighs 1200 ounces submerged in water. What is the specific gravity of the lead?

    A) 0.7
    B) 0.85714
    C) 7
    D) 1.166

4) A calorie is the amount of heat required to raise the temperature of one gram of water _____?

    A) 1 degree F.
    B) 5 degrees K.
    C) 1 degree C.
    D) 5 degrees R.

5) Carry out the following multiplication:
    $$(6.42 \times 10^{-9}) \times (2.58 \times 10^{2})$$
    A) 1.66
    B) 1.66×10^{-4}
    C) 1.66×10^{-5}
    D) 1.66×10^{-6}

6) How many milligrams are there in 0.22 kg?

    A) 2,200,000 mmg

    B) 2.2 g.

    C) 22,000 mg.

    D) 220,000 mg.

7) The three layers of skin are:

    A) Hair follicles, capillary, muscle.

    B) Epidermis, dermis, subcutaneous.

    C) Id, ego, superego.

    D) Cuticle, blood vessel, muscle.

8) If a material with a molecular weight of 90 evaporates from an enclosed process tank, where would it accumulate?

    A) Floor.

    B) Ceiling.

    C) Neither, it will mix uniformly.

    D) Depends on temperature of the material.

9) Which of the following does **not** belong to the halogen family?

    A) Radon.

    B) Chlorine.

    C) Astatine.

    D) Bromine.

10) As one ages, there is a vascular and neural degeneration of the inner ear. This results in a decrease in hearing ability. This condition is called:

    A) Sensorineural.

    B) Sociocusis.

    C) Presbycusis.

    D) Tinnitus.

11) Which of the following chemical equations is balanced?

$$H_2SO_4 + 2NaOH \longrightarrow \quad \text{or} \quad 2AlCl_3 + 3K_2CO_3 \longrightarrow$$

    A) $H_2SO_8 + NaOH_2$

    B) $NaSO + H_4O_4$

    C) $Al(Cl_2) + 3K_3CO_3$

    D) $Al_2(CO_3)_3 + 6KCl$

12) Which of the following does **not** describe the workers' compensation concept of whole-man?

    A) Concept considers functional effects of the loss.
    B) Compares functions after disability with normal fully-functional man.
    C) Disability is rated as a percentage of the whole-man.
    D) Compares actual lost wages compared to potential wages.

13) Which of the following is the permitted worker exposure to ionizing radiation in the United States?

    A) 0.05 rem.
    B) 0.5 rem.
    C) 5 rem.
    D) 4000 millirem.

14) Which of the following **best** describes the audiogram?

    A) An ear-cleaning machine.
    B) A hearing booth and noise measuring instrument.
    C) An indicator of hearing acuity.
    D) A tool to detect high hazard noise areas.

15) A temporary increase in the threshold of hearing is called a:

    A) Occupational Noise Correction Factor (ONCF).
    B) Temporary Threshold Shift (TTS).
    C) Permanent Threshold Shift (PTS).
    D) Reduction Hearing Index (RHI).

16) Which of the following **best** describes the term TLV-STEL?

    A) A concentration that should never be exceeded.
    B) A dose permitted for a 30-minute exposure.
    C) A level generally below the TLV-TWA.
    D) A level for rescue workers.

17) A motorcycle is traveling at 90 mph. The rider's reaction time is 0.7 seconds. How many feet will the motorcycle travel before the rider recognizes an emergency situation and actually applies the brakes?

    A)   132 feet.
    B)   108 feet.
    C)   92.6 feet.
    D)   99.6 feet.

18) The **most common** danger from chromium electroplating is:

    A)   Mists of chromic acid.
    B)   Splashes of acid.
    C)   High Voltage.
    D)   Extremely slippery floors.

19) Toxic materials enter the body through which major routes?

    A)   Inhalation, skin absorption, ingestion.
    B)   Inhalation, capillary absorption, intravenous.
    C)   Inhalation, respiration, breathing.
    D)   Inhalation, skin absorption, eating.

20) Which of the following statements is **not** true about the static pressure in a ventilation system?

    A)   Static Pressure is measured parallel to the direction of flow.
    B)   Static Pressure tends to collapse the duct in an exhaust system.
    C)   Static Pressure acts in all directions.
    D)   Static Pressure is a part of Total Pressure.

21) Workers of which industry are affected by the disease silicosis?

    A)   Government workers.
    B)   Iron workers.
    C)   Coal miners.
    D)   Quartz miners.

22) The majority of hearing loss a OHST will encounter in an industrial setting and caused by industrial exposure is?

    A)   Sensorineural.
    B)   Conductive.
    C)   Osteosclerosis.
    D)   A middle ear problem.

23) Which of the following occupations is **most likely** to contract cumulative trauma disorder?

    A)   Professional who inputs to a computer occasionally.
    B)   Maintenance man.
    C)   Grocery store checkout clerk.
    D)   Auto mechanic who is a tennis player.

24) A locomotive is traveling at 90 mph. The engineer's reaction time is 0.6 seconds. How many feet will the locomotive travel before the engineer recognizes an emergency situation and actually applies the brakes?

    A)   75 feet.
    B)   110 feet.
    C)   80 feet.
    D)   90 feet.

25) Your company has acquired a very high noise vehicle that is operated over the road for extended periods of time. Which piece of equipment would you suggest for monitoring the noise exposure of the vehicle operators?

    A)   Sound level meter.
    B)   Octave band analyzer.
    C)   Noise dosimeter.
    D)   Annual audiogram.

26) When conducting personal air-monitoring using solid-sorbent tube samplers, which of the following instructions apply?

    A)   Tubes should be shaken to prevent packing.
    B)   Tubes should be placed vertically to prevent channeling.
    C)   Tubes should be placed horizontally to prevent channeling.
    D)   Tubes should be shaken to prevent breakthrough.

27) The capacity of a material to produce injury or harm is the definition of which of the following?

 A) Hazard Potential.
 B) Toxicity.
 C) Dangerous Material.
 D) Hazardous Material.

28) A volume of gas is 150 ml at 120 F. What is the volume at 460 degrees R? *Note: $x^\circ R = (t^\circ F) + 460$.

 A) 116.83 ml.
 B) 1168.39 ml.
 C) 118.97 ml.
 D) 188.51 ml.

29) In the study of insurance the term "Risk" is often defined as having two components, that of pure risk and speculative risk? Which of the following is **not** an example of pure risk?

 A) Business failure.
 B) Hail storm.
 C) Liability arising from negligent conduct.
 D) Auto accident with damage & injury.

30) Which of the following correctly indicates the formula for computing WBGT (outdoor)?

 A) WBGT = 0.7 WB + 0.2 GT + 1.0 DB
 B) WBGT = 0.7 WB + 0.3 GT + 5/9 DB
 C) WBGT = 0.7 WB + 0.2 GT + 0.1 DB
 D) WBGT = 0.7 WB + 0.3 GT

31) What is the audible range for an average young person with unimpaired hearing?

 A) Below 20 Hz.
 B) Above 20,000 Hz.
 C) Between 20 - 20,000 Hz.
 D) Between 50 - 30,000 Hz.

32) Which of the following control methods is **least likely** to produce positive results in occupations that have a high potential for cumulative trauma disorders?

    A) Rotation or frequent rest periods.
    B) Substitute machinery to avoid repetitive operations.
    C) Limit fast, hard and extreme movements by any person.
    D) Use Quality Circles - thus allowing the workers to fix the problem.

33) The A-weighted sound level measurement is used as the "standard" scale in occupational noise measurement because:

    A) It weights intermittent and impact noise.
    B) Weighting is related to effects of noise on the ear.
    C) It filters out "white" noise.
    D) It has a built-in dose response curve.

34) Which of the following is **not** correct? Atmospheric pressure is equal to:

    A) 14.7 psi.
    B) 760 mm Hg.
    C) 760 torr.
    D) 111.3 kilopascal.

35) The pH is a measure of a materials acidity or alkalinity. What would a pH of 12 indicate?

    A) A very strong acid.
    B) A basic mixture used for building other compounds.
    C) An alkaline.
    D) A mixture of compounds.

36) What is the minimum level of oxygen required if personnel are to enter a confined space without breathing apparatus?

    A) 19.0%
    B) 17.5%
    C) 19.5%
    D) 16%

37) Which of the following welding processes produces the **most** ultraviolet light?

    A)   Stick welding.
    B)   Oxygen Acetylene welding.
    C)   GAS-shielded welding (argon).
    D)   Laser cutting.

38) Which of the following **best** describes the effect of Carbon Monoxide on the blood?

    A)   Replaces oxygen and reduces white blood cells.
    B)   Replaces oxygen and reduces transportation of oxygen.
    C)   Reduces oxygen capacity of lungs.
    D)   Reduces oxygen in lungs and causes edema.

39) The OSHAct allows individual states to forego OSHA requirements by developing a state plan. These plans must meet certain criteria as set forth by 29 CFR 1904. How long do states have to implement their state plan once OSHA has given its approval?

    A)   30 days.
    B)   3 months.
    C)   1 year.
    D)   3 years.

40) Which law indicates that gases behave consistently with temperature changes?

    A)   Charles' law.
    B)   Boyle's law.
    C)   Newton's law.
    D)   Dalton's law.

41) A body that has a definite volume but no definite shape is?

    A)   A solid.
    B)   A vapor.
    C)   A liquid.
    D)   A fume.

42) What is the maximum travel distance allowed for a fire extinguisher protecting a Light Hazard occupancy?

    A) 75 feet.
    B) 25 feet.
    C) 35 feet.
    D) 50 feet.

43) Which of the following organizations deals with compressed gas cylinder safety?

    A) ANSI.
    B) CGA.
    C) ASTM.
    D) OSHA.

44) A temperature of 50 degrees C equals _____ degrees Kelvin.

    A) 273 degrees.
    B) 373 degrees.
    C) 203 degrees.
    D) 323 degrees.

45) Your company hires a worker unaware of his existing back problem. Three weeks later, this person aggravates his back problem while on the job. Workers' compensation would:

    A) Deny the claim based on ADA.
    B) Pay 100% for a new injury.
    C) Pay only medical expenses and prescriptions.
    D) Deny the claim based on an existing condition.

46) Which of the following are used to adjust Workers' Compensation Insurance Rates?

    A) Experience Modification Rate.
    B) Incident Rate.
    C) Workers' Compensation Mod Rate.
    D) Accident Rate.

47) An audit of safety and health program management has revealed that the program has failed to accomplish the stated objective of accident prevention. Accident rates are very poor, as is morale and discipline. Supervisors openly defy management authority and varying standards exist through the company. Which of the following offers the **best** explanation for the failure of safety program management?

    A) Failure of the safety director to establish an effective program.
    B) Failure of top management to support the accident prevention effort.
    C) Failure of management at all levels to manage, lead and direct the workforce.
    D) Failure of procedures to identify the correct and safe methods for job accomplishment.

48) In order to engender trust, OSHA's VPP approach to applicants is based on all the following principles **except?**

    A) The VPP is strictly voluntary.
    B) During the application process, prior to approval, the application is confidential.
    C) Under the OSH Act, compliance with the provisions of the Act and the standards set under the authority of the Act is mandatory.
    D) VPP participants will work independently to resolve any safety and health problems that may arise during participation.

49) A steel manufacturing plant with a $1,100,000 payroll sustains workers' compensation losses of $90,000 in cy 2003. The experience modification factor for this plant is 1.4 and the manual rate is $7.45 per $100.00 of payroll. What is the modified rate for this company?

    A) $5.53
    B) $7.45
    C) $9.00
    D) $10.43

50) In some combustible gas meters an electrical circuit called the wheatstone bridge circuit is used to measure the mixture of combustible gas to air. Which of the following characteristics concerning this balanced bridge circuit is **not** true?

    A) The presence of a combustible mixture causes catalytic combustion decreasing resistance shown as meter movement.

    B) One leg of the circuit is called a hot wire.

    C) The platinum element can be poisoned by small amounts of silicone.

    D) The hot wire detector requires oxygen to function.

51) There is a 2000 gallon tank filled with brine water (s.g. 1.8). What will be the weight of a full tank?

    A) 16,800 lbs.

    B) 26,900 lbs.

    C) 30,000 lbs.

    D) 40,000 lbs.

52) In some industrial occupancies, fire doors are provided to allow compartmentalization of the facility and prevent the spread of fire and smoke. If these doors are equipped with self-closing devices they must be inspected regularly to assure operation. All of the following are valid inspection items **except?**

    A) Check lubrication on guides and bearings.

    B) Check to insure fusible links are painted to prevent rust.

    C) Check binders are not bent, thus obstructing the door.

    D) Check to insure chains or wire ropes have not stretched.

53) Your company has a cutting area with 5 identical machines. The noise is monitored at 97 dB. If 4 machines were removed from the area, what would you expect for the new noise measurement?

    A) 90 dB.

    B) 92 dB.

    C) 97 dB.

    D) 104 dB.

54) Before installation, abrasive wheels should be inspected and tested. One accepted type of testing is called a _____ test.
- A) Sounding.
- B) Ring.
- C) Speed.
- D) Roundness.

55) Which of the following is **not** a recognized class of protective footwear?
- A) Conductive shoes/boots.
- B) Foundry shoes.
- C) Safety-Toe Safety Shoes Class "75".
- D) Non-ionizing, worker Safety Shoe Class "EX" radiation.

56) The "Zero Mechanical State" principle of guarding is generally understood to mean?
- A) All energy sources are neutralized.
- B) All electrical energy is off.
- C) Guards are in a zero or down position.
- D) The machine is not operational (Zero Mechanical State).

57) The **primary** reason for enclosing a grinding wheel is:
- A) Maintain collection system.
- B) Contain parts of the wheel should breakage occur.
- C) Support tool rest.
- D) Prevent wheel from breaking.

58) Warning signs, hazardous material labels and other forms of warnings must be in:
- A) English.
- B) English and Spanish.
- C) All the languages spoken in a workplace.
- D) The standard does not specify the language.

59) The volume of 1 g-mole of nitrogen at 760 mm Hg and 25°C is:
- A) 14.0 liters.
- B) 24.5 liters.
- C) 22.4 liters.
- D) 44.4 liters.

60) How much air is required for workers performing sand-blasting operation and equipped with Type-C supplied-air hoods?
   A) 3 CFM.
   B) 6 CFM.
   C) 9 CFM.
   D) 12 CFM.

61) Acclimatization to heat is generally achieved by requiring the employee to?
   A) Work at 50% of the desired work rate.
   B) Work at 75% of the desired work rate.
   C) Work for two hours per day for two weeks.
   D) Work for six hours per day for two months.

62) Which of the following **best** defines the operation of a rate of rise heat detector?
   A) Detects heat and signals an alarm.
   B) Detects the speed of a temperature rise.
   C) Detects the amount of temperature rise.
   D) Detects the radiant energy of combustibles.

63) Which of the following **best** describes the science of kinematics?
   A) Dealing with force.
   B) Dealing with time.
   C) Dealing with spatial relationships.
   D) Dealing with motion.

64) Which of the following is **not** true concerning the electrical Ground Fault Circuit Interrupter?
   A) It requires an equipment ground to function.
   B) It is a very fast acting device.
   C) It will not detect line-to-line faults.
   D) It is designed for personnel protection.

65) Which of the following is the **most effective** way of reducing the effects of radiant heat on the occupational employee?
   A) A minimum of 15 room changes of air per hour.
   B) Blow cool air on employee.
   C) Provide shielding.
   D) Provide worker with layers of clothing.

66) All of the following statements concerning combustible gas indicators (CGIs) are true **except?**
   A)   CGIs will work in areas with very little oxygen.
   B)   CGIs can be used on a wide variety of gases.
   C)   Most CGIs work on the principle of heat of combustion.
   D)   CGIs are direct reading instruments.

67) General or dilution ventilation is **not** appropriate in which of the following situations?
   A)   When small quantities of contaminants are released.
   B)   The toxicity of contaminants is low.
   C)   Air is drawn through the workers' breathing zone.
   D)   The operation is of low duration and frequency.

68) A needs assessment does all the following **except?**
   A)   Identifies the type of training required.
   B)   Identifies the problem or need before designing a solution.
   C)   Saves time and money by ensuring that solutions effectively address the problems they are intended to solve.
   D)   Identifies factors that will impact the training before its development.

69) You make face velocity readings over equal areas on a fully open exhaust hood with an opening of 3 feet by 3 feet. The measurements are 80 fpm, 115 fpm, 125 fpm and 100 fpm. What is the airflow in cfm?
   A)   850.
   B)   900.
   C)   945.
   D)   1125.

70) What organization has established the TLVs used in industry today?
   A)   MSHA.
   B)   ACGIH.
   C)   EPA.
   D)   Dept. of Health.

71) Which of the following ANSI Standards deal with Safety Glasses?

    A)   ANSI Z16.1
    B)   ANSI A17.1
    C)   ANSI Z87.1
    D)   ANSI Z89.1

72) The vehicle operator of a commercial truck must conform with the requirements of what agency when operating within the confines of the United States?

    A)   DOT.
    B)   OSHA.
    C)   EPA.
    D)   FHA.

73) If a person is suffering from heatstroke, which symptom would they **not** experience?

    A)   Severe headache.
    B)   Profuse sweating and cool moist skin.
    C)   Loss of consciousness.
    D)   Rapid temperature rise and hot dry skin.

74) Which of the following is the **most frequent** cause of occupational dermatosis?

    A)   Alkaline soaps.
    B)   Hand creams.
    C)   Water based solvents.
    D)   Acids and Alkalis.

75) Which of the following provides the **best** reason for providing an electrical equipment ground wire on an electrical branch circuit?

    A)   Provide a low resistance path for fault currents.
    B)   Provide a path for line-to-line problems.
    C)   Provide a counterpoise to insure both wires are balanced.
    D)   Ensure that an extra neutral is available in case the black wire breaks.

76) In which of the following instances would it be permissible to connect a separate electrical ground wire to the case of a portable appliance, rather than using a properly connected three wire power cord?

    A) Anytime, normal practice.
    B) In an emergency.
    C) Only if the circuit was protected by a circuit breaker.
    D) If a GFI was used.

77) What type of respirator protection would you recommend for employees working in the layup area of a fiberglass manufacturing facility?

    A) Mechanical Filter.
    B) Supplied air.
    C) Chemical Cartridge.
    D) Self-Contained Breathing Air.

78) Which of the following **best** describes a Class "A" level of Personal Protective Equipment (PPE)?

    A) Fully-encapsulated chemical-resistant suit with Self Contained Breathing Apparatus (SCBA) or Supplied Air (SA) with escape provisions.
    B) Chemical-resistant suit with Self Contained Breathing Apparatus (SCBA) or Supplied Air (SA) with escape provisions.
    C) Chemical-resistant suit with Air Purifying Respirator (APR).
    D) No chemical protection and no respiratory protection.

79) Under which of the following categories would a noise-induced hearing loss be recorded on the OSHA 300 Log?

    A) Injury.
    B) Skin Disorder.
    C) All Other Illnesses.
    D) Hearing Loss.

Five year mishap history "ABC" Corporation

Year	Total Recordable Columns G, H I, J	LWDs	LWD Cases Columns H & I	Days Away from Work	Days of Restricted Work Activity	hours
2006	92	1932	67	1565	367	1,398,765
2007	88	2002	81	1622	380	1,456,732
2008	119	1821	98	1384	137	1,129,565
2009	118	1754	90	1316	438	1,623,451
2010	122	1234	98	740	494	1,834,225

80) Given the information in the accident information chart shown above, determine the DART rate for 2009.

   A) 2.16
   B) 27.6
   C) 11.1
   D) 9.01

81) Determine the recordable accident rate for the last three years shown in the chart used in the preceding question.

   A) 15.7
   B) 11.8
   C) 31.4
   D) 2.76

82) Determine the cumulative DART accident rate for the 5 years shown in the chart used in the preceding question.

   A) 27.7
   B) 2.76
   C) 10.9
   D) 11.7

83) Which of the following would most likely **not** be included in a lesson plan developed for a Health and Safety Training Session?

   A) Introduction.
   B) Objectives.
   C) Training Aids.
   D) Student Survey.

84) Which of the following is the **most often recommended** fundamental safety training for plant workers?

   A)   First Aid, Supervisor's Safety, and Welding.
   B)   Welding, Forktruck Training, and Back-Care.
   C)   Fire Extinguisher Training, First Aid, and Contingency.
   D)   Contingency, First Aid, and Vehicle Operations.

85) Which of the following is **not** a purpose for displaying safety posters?

   A)   As a substitute for management support.
   B)   To remind of specific hazards.
   C)   Maintain a high level of safety awareness.
   D)   To provide instructions on safety equipment.

86) Which of the following is in the **best** position to provide effective safety training of industrial work groups?

   A)   Supervisors.
   B)   Senior Management.
   C)   OHSTs.
   D)   Training Professionals.

87) The term "incident rate" is used quite often in the expanding field of safety and health. In industrial safety work the term is most commonly associated with minor mishaps or the frequency of all mishaps. In epidemiology, the term incidence rate is often used to indicate the number of _____ that occurred in a given period of time.

   A)   New cases.
   B)   Prevalent cases.
   C)   All cases.
   D)   Specific cases.

88) Which of the following training methods is primarily used to find new, innovative approaches to issues?

   A)   Meeting.
   B)   Brainstorming.
   C)   Case Study.
   D)   Role Playing.

89) Safety and health training can involve many different delivery systems and training techniques. Often group methods are used to increase the effectiveness of training and the active participation by students. Which of the following would be the **best** use of the role-playing technique?

    A) In human relations training.
    B) For job instruction training in a one-on-one situation.
    C) To illustrate the complexities of a step-by-step detailed industrial task.
    D) For in-depth technical subjects.

90) The OSHA DART is frequently used in industrial safety work. This indicator should be used as:

    A) An absolute rate to compare with other industries.
    B) An indicator of serious injury frequency.
    C) A yardstick after converting to a million manhours.
    D) An accident severity rate to compare your severity and frequency against other similar industry rates.

91) Which of the following is true concerning the electrical Ground Fault Circuit Interrupter?

    A) It requires an equipment ground to function.
    B) It is a very slow acting device.
    C) It will not detect line-to-line faults.
    D) It is not designed for personnel protection.

92) Fuel and oxygen cylinders in storage locations must be separated by a minimum distance, or a firewall must be provided. If a firewall is provided the fire resistance rating of the wall must be at least?

    A) ½ hour.
    B) 1 hour.
    C) 2 hours.
    D) 3 hours.

93) During the establishment of the company lockout-tagout program you have trained employees, provided locks and tags, and developed a generic general purpose servicing procedure. You have had no accidents involving the unexpected activation or re-energization of machines or equipment during the last 10 years. Under which of the following situations could you still be cited by OSHA under the requirements in 1910.147?

    A)   There are no equipment or machines with stored energy.
    B)   Locks used for lock-out are color coded red.
    C)   Tags do not have employee pictures.
    D)   Several machines have multiple energy sources.

94) The Fire Protection Handbook is published by which of the following organizations?

    A)   OSHA.
    B)   NIOSH.
    C)   NSC.
    D)   NFPA.

95) You are transiting the production area and spot a safety hazard that presents imminent danger to the workers in the area. Your first action should be to:

    A)   Shut down the production line.
    B)   Fix the hazard.
    C)   Post a lock-out/tag-out sign until the hazard is corrected.
    D)   Notify the area supervisor to get the hazard corrected.

96) In order to provide a safe work place, the safety professional should:

    A)   Always seek an outside opinion before making a decision.
    B)   Consult the local ASSE chapter for guidance when needed.
    C)   Make decisions on all situations based on their knowledge.
    D)   Limit their advice and recommendation to those areas that they have knowledge in.

97) Once you obtained your OHST, you must maintain your currency in the safety and health arena. This is monitored by the BCSP by the Certification Maintenance program. If you fail to meet your required 20 points in five years, you must:

   A) Obtain 50 points in the next five-year period.
   B) Complete 20 college credits to be reinstated.
   C) Retake the OHST exam.
   D) Resubmit an application for reevaluation.

98) You are conducting a safety inspection of a manufacturing plant in the southwest. The inspection is designed to fulfill two purposes, one to indoctrinate a new junior safety engineer, and second to uncover non-compliance with federal, state and local directives. During your inspection you observe an employee, without eye protection, working at a bench installing parts. This is not a hazardous operation but it is a posted "eye protection" area. Which of the following is the **best** course of action?

   A) Contact the supervisor and discuss the situation.
   B) Test the junior safety engineer's skills by letting her handle the situation.
   C) Confront the employee and determine "Why" eye protection is not being used.
   D) Note the discrepancy and do not discuss it until the out brief when the CEO and the supervisor are both present.

99) Which of the following key label elements are standardized under the Globally Harmonized System (GHS)?

   A) Product identifier, Supplier identifier, Chemical identity.
   B) Hazard pictograms, Signal words, Hazard statements.
   C) Precautionary information, Product identifier, Hazard statements.
   D) Signal words, Chemical identity, Hazard pictograms.

100) For protection against chlorinated solvents and jobs requiring dexterity and sensitivity, which type of chemical-resistant gloves are preferred?

   A) Butyl.
   B) Neoprene.
   C) Nitrile.
   D) Polyvinyl alcohol (PVA).

Self-Assessment Exam One Answers

1) We selected answer B because:

Anhydrous means without water.

2) We selected answer B because:

pH = -log [H+] pH equals minus the logarithm of the hydrogen ion concentration in moles per liter. Using the calculator, $-\text{Log}(2.3 \times 10^{-5})$ = 4.64. The pH scale extends from 0 to 14, values less than 7 are acids and greater than 7 are bases.

3) We selected answer C because:

Specific gravity is the ratio of the weight's weight to an equal mass of water. SG=ds/dw; where d=w/v. Since the difference in weight on land and in the water is 200 ounces, then an amount of water the same density as the weight must weigh 200 ounces, but the lead weighs 1400 ounces so 1400÷200 = 7 times heavier than water. SG = 7.

4) We selected answer C because:

The calorie is the amount of heat required to raise the temperature of one gram of water one degree Celsius.

5) We selected answer D because:

Multiply decimal numerals. Add exponents & you get:

6.42 × 2.58 = 16.6   -9 + 2 = -7

$16.6 \times 10^{-7} = 1.66 \times 10^{-6}$

6) We selected answer D because:

$$\frac{0.22 \text{ kg}}{1} \times \frac{1000 \text{ g}}{1 \text{ kg}} \times \frac{1000 \text{ mg}}{1 \text{ g}} = 220,000 \text{ mg}$$

7) We selected answer B because:

The 3 layers of the skin are the epidermis (outer-layer) the dermis (true skin) and the subcutaneous tissue.

8) We selected answer A because:

Determining where gases will accumulate is a complicated subject because of the tendency of the gas to be dispersed by air movement. However, the best answer to this question is that the gas will sink to the floor given the Molecular Weight *(MW)* of 90 (very heavy). Air has a MW of about 30. The National Fire Protection Association Fire Protection Handbook has additional information.

9) We selected answer A because:

Radon is the obvious and correct choice.

10) We selected answer C because:

Presbycusis is hearing loss due to the normal process of aging. *Sociocusis* refers to hearing loss due to non-occupational noise sources such as: household noise, tv, radio, traffic etc. *Tinnitus* is ringing in the ears. *Sensorineural* is loss of hearing due to occupational exposure.

11) We selected answer D because:

This equation is the only one balanced.

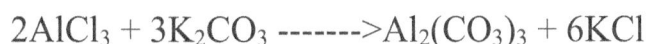

$$2AlCl_3 + 3K_2CO_3 \text{ -------} > Al_2(CO_3)_3 + 6KCl$$

Because, both sides [$2AlCl_3 + 3K_2CO_3$ & $Al_2(CO_3)_3 + 6KCl$] have:

Two (2) Aluminum (Al) atoms,
Six (6) Chlorine (Cl) atoms,
Six (6) Potassium (K) atoms,
Three (3) Carbon (C) atoms,
Nine (9) Oxygen (O) atoms

12) We selected answer D because:

The whole-man theory compares the function of a whole unimpaired man with the ability to function after a disabling injury. The disability is rated in percentage and then compared to the income potential. Answer D more appropriately describes the concept of "Lost Wages" which considers the reduction in earnings that was caused by the accident compared to a standard that approximates what the worker would have earned if uninjured. The compensation attempts to make up the difference.

13) We selected answer C because:

The limit for ionizing radiation in the United States, is established by the Nuclear Regulatory Commission, at 5 rem per year.

14) We selected answer C because:

An audiogram is a record of hearing loss or hearing level measured at several different frequencies, normally from 500 to 6000 hertz. Hearing levels are generally presented graphically as a function of frequency. The audiogram measures the acuity or sharpness of hearing ability.

15) We selected answer B because:

A temporary depression of the hearing is called a Temporary Threshold Shift or TTS. When people are exposed to a high level of noise, they almost always exhibit a transient attenuation in their ability to hear. This *temporary threshold shift* (TTS) usually vanishes a few hours after the exposure. One theory has held that a *permanent threshold shift* (PTS) is simply the result of a large number of TTSs', each superimposed on the last. According to that theory, avoidance of any demonstrable TTS should result in no PTS.

16) We selected answer A because:

The 1989-1990 Threshold Limit Values and Biological Exposure Indices Booklet TLV book states: "A STEL is defined as a 15-minute TWA exposure which should not be exceeded at any time during a work day even if the 8-hour TWA is within the TLV-TWA. Exposures above the TLV-TWA up to the STEL should not be longer than 15 minutes and should not occur more than four times per day. There should be at least 60 minutes between successive exposures in this range. An averaging period other than 15 minutes may be recommended when this is warranted by observed biological effects."

17) We selected answer C because:

Distance = Speed times Time.

$$D = \frac{(90 \times 5280)}{(60 \times 60)} \times 0.7 \text{ seconds}$$

$$D = 92.6 \text{ feet}$$

HINT: 5280÷3600 = 1.47 (a constant that is often used in these type of problems) 1.47 times MPH = feet per second

$$90 \times 1.47 \times 0.7 = 92.6$$

18) We selected answer A because:

The most common and most damaging hazard in chrome electroplating is inhalation of the chromic acid mists.

19) We selected answer A because:

The most common ways for toxic materials to enter the body is through the skin by absorption, by inhalation and through ingestion.

20)   We selected answer A because:

Static pressure is always measured perpendicular to the direction of flow.

21)   We selected answer D because:

Quartz miners would be exposed to the fine quartz dust that can cause silicosis.

22)   We selected answer A because:

Most industrial exposure is sensorineural or noise induced.

23)   We selected answer C because:

Cumulative trauma disorders involve repeated use of a body part. They normally surface as carpal tunnel syndrome, tarsal tunnel syndrome, tendinitis, bursitis, and tenosynovitis. In this question any of the activities cited have the potential for cumulative trauma disorder. However, the most likely choice is that of checkout clerk because the job requires repetitive and prolonged extreme wrist movement.

24)   We selected answer C because:

Distance = Speed times Time.

$$D = \frac{(90 \times 5280)}{(60 \times 60)} \times 0.6 \text{ seconds}$$

HINT: $5280 \div 3600 = 1.47$ (a constant that is often used in these type of problems) 1.47 times MPH = feet per second

$D = 79.2$ feet

$$90 \times 1.47 \times 0.6 = 79.4 \text{ feet}$$

25)   We selected answer C because:

Sound level meters would require constant readings and a technician to note the readings. The same holds true for *octave band analysis. Annual audiograms* are, of course, an after the fact measure. *Noise dosimeters* would be easy to use and would provide the measurement desired in this case.

26)   We selected answer B because:

When conducting personal sampling using solid sorbent, eg: charcoal silica gel, porous polymers etc. the tube should be positioned vertically during sampling to avoid channeling and premature breakthrough.

27)   We selected answer B because:

According to the National Safety Council, "Toxicity is the capacity of a material to produce injury or harm". This differs considerably for the classic definition of hazard, which is the possibility that exposure to a material can cause injury or illness.

28)   We selected answer C because:

$$\frac{P_1 V_1}{T_1} = \frac{P_2 V_2}{T_2}$$

$$\frac{150}{580} = \frac{V_2}{460}$$

$$V_2 = \frac{150 \times 460}{580} = 118.97 \ mL$$

29) We selected answer A because:

In insurance terms "Risk" is usually separated into two entities, pure risk and speculative risk. *Pure risk* implies two outcomes ie; fiscal loss or no fiscal loss. The choices are, to have a loss or not to have a loss, however there is no choice that could be considered a gain. To have a loss is certainly not a gain, and to not have a loss is neutral. Pure risk is generally divided into personal and property. *Speculative loss* implies three choices; loss, no loss, or gain. Speculation in the stock market implies three choices: the stock goes up (gain), the stock goes down (loss), and the stock remains the same (neutral). Speculative risks are sometimes called business risks. The distinction is made in the study of insurance to illustrate the concept that only rarely is insurance applied to speculative risk. Most all insurance attempts to protect one from the misfortune of loss, that is, pure risk.

30) We selected answer C because:

The formula for computing WBGT is listed in the Formulae, Equations, Constants, and Conversions sheet issued during the test.

$$WBGT = 0.7\ WB + 0.2\ GT + 0.1\ DB$$

31) We selected answer C because:

Below 20 Hz is sub-audible, above 20,000 is ultrasonic. The average measured hearing range of an unimpaired person is 20-20,000 Hz.

32) We selected answer D because:

All of the selections have the potential for solving the cause of cumulative trauma disorders, that is, repeated use of the hand or other body part. However, many times the workers themselves are not in the best position to judge which actions can cause body stress. Additionally, not all people are equally susceptible to these types of injuries making it difficult for a group of people to agree on the root cause. We think in this case "Quality Circles" have the least chance to solve this problem.

33) We selected answer B because:

   The A-weighting most closely weights the sound to the injurious effects of the noise on the ear.

34) We selected answer D because:

   Atmospheric pressure is equal to 14.7 psi or 760 mm Hg or 760 torr or **101.3 kilopascal.**

35) We selected answer C because:

   The pH is a number that indicates the acidity or alkalinity of an aqueous solution. The range of the pH scale is from 0 to 14. Aqueous solutions having a pH from 0 to 7 are *acidic*. Aqueous solutions having a pH from 7 to 14 are basic, or caustic, or alkaline. A material having a pH of 12 would be an alkaline.

36) We selected answer C because:

   According to OSHA a minimum of 19.5% oxygen content is required before entry into a confined space is allowed without the use of supplied air.

37) We selected answer C because:

   Gas-shielded welding generates extremely high amounts of ultraviolet radiation. A typical application, using a shield of argon gas around the arc doubles the intensity of the ultraviolet radiation. The use of increased currents with a consumable electrode will increase the production of ultraviolet to as great as thirty times the exposure with a non-shielded operation.

38) We selected answer B because:

   Carbon Monoxide has about 250 times the affinity of oxygen for the hemoglobin and thus greatly reduces transportation of oxygen.

39) We selected answer D because:

29 CFR 1902.1(c)(1) requires that a state have its plan implemented within 3 years of its approval by OSHA.

1902.3(c)(1)

The State plan shall include or provide for the development or adoption of, and contain assurances that the State will continue to develop or adopt, standards which are or will be at least as effective as those promulgated under section 6 of the Act.

This means that it must at least cover everything in 29 CFR 1910, but the state can add additional areas.

40) We selected answer A because:

Gases behave consistently with temperature changes. This is stated in Charles's Law: At a constant pressure the volume of a confined gas varies directly as the absolute temperature; and at a constant volume, the pressure varies directly as the absolute temperature. NOTE: The use of absolute temperature!

41) We selected answer C because:

A liquid has no definite shape but a definite volume.

42) We selected answer A because:

The maximum travel distance to a fire extinguisher regardless of the rating for Class A hazards is 75 feet.

43) We selected answer B because:

The CGA (Compressed Gas Association) as the name indicates is the primary organization dealing with compressed gas safety in the U. S.

44) We selected answer D because:

To convert t_c to t_K you must add 273.16

$$50 + 273 = 323$$

45) We selected answer B because:

Since the company did not know about the existing problem and it was not documented, this would be treated as a new injury.

46) We selected answer A because:

The insurance industry uses EMR for workers' compensation insurance as a means of determining equitable premiums. These rating systems consider the average incident losses for a given firm's type of work and amount of payroll and predict the dollar amount of expected losses due to work-related injuries and illnesses.

All 50 states, DC, Guam and Puerto Rico have worker's compensation laws. If you have an experience modifier greater than 1, you have above average losses and a less than standard performance. The EMR is based on the last 3 years loss history, not including the previous year.

47) We selected answer C because:

Safety and the responsibility for achieving it rests with management, primarily with the organization's chief executive officer, but in a shared manner with all other managers. There has always been disagreement in management circles about just how to accomplish safety, but there has always been agreement that management of safety, like all other functions has to start at the top, and be supported by subordinate executives and managers. Supervisors, foremen and workers develop their attitude about the importance of safety & health from both formal and informal clues. A divided position by management sends a clue that management is really not all that interested in safety and it's just another one of those things they have to say. Management of the safety and health effort is both an art and a science and the Director of Safety & Health is merely the steward of the function. When safety is effective, the entire management team deserves the credit, likewise when it fails the entire team deserves the blame.

However, the first-line supervisors are the one's primarily responsible for implementing and enforcing the company's loss control and safety and health programs.

48) We selected answer D because:

According to the **VPP Philosophy,** the VPP approach to applicants is based on the following principles:

- Voluntarism
- Confidentiality
- Compliance and Beyond
- Hazard Prevention
- Cooperation - VPP staff and approved VPP participants will work together to resolve any safety and health problems that may arise during participation.

The program consists of four major elements, management commitment, work site analysis, hazard prevention & control and safety & health training.

Injury and Illness History Requirements. Injury and illness history at the site is evaluated using a 3-year total case incident rate (TCIR) and a 3-year day away, restricted, and/or transfer case incident rate (DART rate). (See Appendix A.) The 3-year TCIR and DART rates must be compared to the most recently published Bureau of Labor Statistics (BLS) national average for the three or four-digit (if available) Standard Industrial Classification code (SIC). The TCIR and DART rates must be compared to the five- or six-digit North American Industrial Classification System (NAICS) code for the industry in which the applicant is classified when the NAICS system is adopted. The BLS publishes SIC and NAICS industry averages 2 years after data is collected. (For example, in calendar year 2003, calendar year 2001 national averages will be available and used for comparison).

Both the 3-year TCIR and the 3-year DART rate must be below the most recently published BLS national average for the specific SIC or NAICS code.

The requirement for a Star sight to have a 3-year injury and illness rate that is below their respective industry is to be modified such that an applicant/participant's rate must be below their respective industries injury and illness rate plus 10%. As a result a Star worksite may have an injury and illness rate above the national average if it is within 10% of that BLS average.

49) We selected answer D because:

$$\text{Modified Rate} = \text{Manual Rate} \times \text{EM}$$

$$7.45 \times 1.4 = 10.43$$

50) We selected answer A because:

Selection "A" is not true. The presence of a combustible mixture causes catalytic combustion on the surface of the hot wire causing an increase in resistance that is converted into a meter movement. The other characteristics of the combustible gas analyzer and the wheatstone bridge circuit are true.

51) We selected answer C because:

Brine is a solution of water and salt. It can be salt water, pickling water, sea water, etc. All forms of brine are heavier than water.

Step 1:	Use conversion for calculating weight of tank containing water.	$2000 \,\text{gal} \times 8.43 \,\text{lbs/gal} = 16{,}680 \,\text{lbs}$
Step 2:	Convert from water to brine using specific gravity.	$16{,}680 \,\text{lbs} \times 1.8 = 30{,}024 \,\text{lbs}$

52) We selected answer B because:

Fusible lead links should not be painted because the paint affects the temperature at which the links will melt.

The best source for data on testing and certifying or approving fire-rated doors is Factory Mutual Global (FM Global).

53) We selected answer A because:

Step 1: Select formula for sources and solve.

$$L_w = 10 \times \log_{10}\left[\frac{W}{W_0}\right]$$

$$L_w = 10 \times \log\left[\frac{1}{5}\right]$$

$$L_w = -7\text{dB}$$

Step 2: Add result to initial reading.

$$dB = 97 + -7$$

$$dB = 90$$

54) We selected answer B because:

Wheels should be given a "ring" test before installation. This test consists of freely suspending the wheel and tapping it lightly with a wooden dowel. A good wheel will render a clear ring and a bad or cracked wheel will sound flat or hollow.

55) We selected answer D because:

There is not a category of protective footwear designed especially for Non-ionizing radiation workers. *Conductive footwear* offering a resistance below 450k OHMs is available to allow for dissipation of static charges. Typical applications would include some types of munitions manufacturing, cleaning tanks that have contained flammable liquids, etc. The *ANSI Std. Z41 "Safety-Toe Footwear"* groups Safety Toe Footwear into three classes which indicates the impact weight the shoes are designed to withstand while maintaining a 16/32 (15/32 for women) inch clearance inside the shoe. The classes are 75, 50 and 30. *Foundry shoes* often have no fasteners that enable quick removal and are used where workers are subject to splashes of molten metal.

56)   We selected answer D because:

Zero Mechanical State (ZMS) is a common term used in ANSI, OSHA, and other well recognized safety literature. The term implies that all energy sources have been depleted. That is, there is no potential energy available to cause harm.

57)   We selected answer B because:

The primary reason for installing full enclosure guards on grinding wheels is to contain pieces of the wheel should it break during operation.

58)   We selected answer A because:

OSHA 29 CFR 1910.1200 requires that all information be presented in English (other languages can be used in addition to English).

59)   We selected answer B because:

From the Formula, Equations, Constants, and Conversions issued at the examination by the testing service and included in the Candidate Handbook, the volume of 1 mole of any gas at 25°C and 1 atm of pressure is 24.5 liters.

60)   We selected answer B because:

To create a positive pressure and allow enough air for breathing at least 6 CFM must be provided each loose-fitting helmet or hood.

61)   We selected answer C because:

Acclimatization to heat is generally achieved by having the employee exposed to the hot environment for two hours per day for one or two weeks.

62)   We selected answer B because:

The rate of rise heat detector, as the name implies, detects a rapid rise in temperature and activates, normally triggering an alarm or suppression unit.

63)   We selected answer D because:

Kinematics is defined as the branch of mechanics dealing with pure motion, without reference to the masses or forces involved.

64)   We selected answer A because:

The Ground-Fault Circuit Interrupter is a fast-action device, which senses a small current leakage to ground and, in a fraction of a second, shuts off the electricity and *interrupts* the faulty flow to ground. Placed between the electrical service and the tool or appliance it serves, the GFCI continually monitors the amount of current going to and from the tool along the normal path of the circuit conductors. Whenever the amount *going* differs from the amount *returning* by a set trip level the GFCI interrupts the electric power within 1/40th of a second. This difference in current is called leakage current to ground and the path it takes to ground could be through a person - in which case, the rapid response of the GFCI is fast enough to prevent electrocution. This protection provided by the GFCI is independent of the condition of the equipment grounding conductor, thus, the GFCI can provide protection even if the equipment grounding conductor becomes inoperative. However, It will not detect line-to-line faults.

65)   We selected answer C because:

Shielding is an effective counter measure against the effects of radiant heat. To be most effective the material used for shielding should be shiny and reflective. Non-reflective metal is not used because it tends to act as a "black body" that absorbs heat and then reradiates heat as a secondary source of radiation. Ventilation has no noticeable effect on radiant heat transfer.

66) We selected answer A because:

The first statement is false. Combustible Gas Indicators (CGIs) cannot function in an oxygen deficient atmosphere, this is one of the major drawbacks when using this instrument. However, Combustible Gas Indicators (CGIs) can be used to detect a wide variety of gases. Normally the meter is calibrated for methane and adjustments to the reading for the gas you wish must be made. The third statement is, of course, true most CGIs are of the hot-wire type and work on the principle of heat of combustion. Combustible Gas Indicators (CGIs) are direct reading instruments.

67) We selected answer C because:

Dilution ventilation is generally restricted to the following conditions:

- Small quantities of contaminant are released into the workplace air and at fairly uniform rates.

- The workplace contaminants are of low toxicity.

- Dilution ventilation will not cause corrosion or damage to equipment in the work area.

- There is enough room to allow air movement to dilute the contaminant to a low level.

- Dilution air can be discharged to the atmosphere without causing community environmental concerns.

68) We selected answer A because:

According to the NSC, a needs assessment helps to:

- Distinguishes between training and non-training needs

- Identifies the problem or need before designing a solution
- Saves time and money by ensuring that solutions effectively address the problems they are intended to solve
- Identifies factors that will impact the training before its development

After the needs assessment, training goals are developed and during that process you will determine what knowledge the trainee needs to know to eliminate the problem. Remember, if you want them to tell time, then teach them how to tell time, not how to build a watch.

69) We selected answer C because:

$$\text{Average Velocity} = \frac{80\ \text{fpm} + 115\ \text{fpm} + 125\ \text{fpm} + 100\ \text{fpm}}{4} = 105\ \text{fpm}$$

$$\text{Area} = 3\ \text{ft} \times 3\ \text{ft} = 9\ \text{ft}^2$$

$$Q = AV$$

$$Q = 9 \times 105 = 945\ \text{cfm}$$

70) We selected answer B because:

The American Conference of Governmental Industrial Hygienists establishes the TLV commonly in use today. OSHA recently has also established some limit values that are Permissible Exposure Limits (PEL).

71) We selected answer C because:

ANSI Z87.1 "Practice for Occupational and Educational Eye and Face Protection." ANSI Z16.1 "Method of Recording and Measuring Work Injury Experience." ANSI A17.1 "Elevators, Escalators, and Moving Walks." ANSI Z89.1 "Protective Headware for Industrial Workers."

72)   We selected answer A because:

The Department of Transportation governs trucking regulations and rules.

73)   We selected answer B because:

During heatstroke (sunstroke) the body temperature rises and reaches a point where the heat-regulating mechanism breaks down completely. The body temperature then rises rapidly. The symptoms are hot dry skin, severe headache, visual disturbances, rapid temperature rise, and loss of consciousness.

74)   We selected answer D because:

Acids and alkalis are involved in a substantial amount of the total reported cases of occupational dermatitis.

75)   We selected answer A because:

The purpose of an electrical equipment ground is to provide a low resistance path for ground faults. This allows the circuit breaker to function and provide protection from electrocution.

76)   We selected answer B because:

Grounding of portable tools, appliances, equipment etc. is normally accomplished by means of a separate green insulated equipment grounding conductor carried with the current carrying conductors in the power cord. Use of a separate external grounding conductor is not desirable because of the impedance developed in a separate external conductor. However, in an emergency it would be permissible if protected from physical damage.

77)   We selected answer A because:

The layup area of a fiberglass facility would most likely contain fibers and dust thus the logical filter would be a mechanical particulate matter.

78) We selected answer A because:

Levels	Skin	Respiratory	When
Modified Chart of EPA/OSHA Levels of Protection			
A	Fully-encapsulating, chemical-resistant suit, inner gloves, chemical-resistant safety boots.	Pressure-demand, full-facepiece SCBA or pressure-demand supplied-air respirator with escape SCBA.	Highest level of protection indicated by high concentration of atmospheric vapors, gases or particulates or splash hazard exists.
B	Chemical-resistant clothing (overalls and long-sleeved jacket; hooded, one or two piece chemical splash suit; disposable chemical-resistant one-piece suit), inner and outer gloves, chemical resistant safety boots and hard hat.	Pressure-demand, full-facepiece SCBA or pressure-demand supplied-air respirator with escape SCBA.	High level of respiratory protection required, but less skin protection. IDLH, less than 19.5% oxygen.
C	Chemical-resistant clothing (overalls and long-sleeved jacket; hooded, one or two piece chemical splash suit; disposable chemical-resistant one-piece suit), inner and outer gloves, chemical resistant safety boots and hard hat.	Full-facepiece, air-purifying, canister-equipped respirator.	The contaminants, splashes, or direct contact will not affect exposed flesh. Canister will remove contaminant.
D	Overalls, Safety Boots, safety glasses or chemical splash goggles, hardhat.	No respiratory protection and minimal skin protection.	The atmosphere contains no known hazard. Splashes, immersion or inhalation improbable

79) We selected answer D because:

Recordable occupational illnesses on the OSHA 300 log are categorized as follows:

- Illnesses
- Skin disorder
- Respiratory condition
- Poisoning
- Hearing Loss
- All other illnesses

80)   We selected answer C because:

$$\text{Rate} = \frac{\text{H \& I Recordables} \times 200{,}000}{\text{Total hours worked}}$$

$$\text{Rate} = \frac{90 \times 200{,}000}{1{,}623{,}451}$$

$$\text{Rate} = \frac{18{,}000{,}000}{1{,}623{,}451}$$

$$\text{Rate} = 11.1$$

81)   We selected answer A because:

Step 1:	Total the number of accidents for the period in question.	119
		118
		122
		359

Step 2:	Total manhours for the same period.	1,129,565
		1,623,451
		1,834,225
		4,587,241

Step 3:   Apply the formula and compute the cumulative accident rate.

$$\text{Rate} = \frac{\text{Total Recordables} \times 200{,}000}{\text{Total hours worked}}$$

$$\text{Rate} = \frac{359 \times 200{,}000}{4{,}587{,}241}$$

$$\text{Rate} = \frac{71{,}800{,}000}{4{,}587{,}241}$$

$$\text{Rate} = 15.7$$

82)   We selected answer D because:

Step 1:	Total the number of accidents for the period in question.	67
		81
		98
		90
		98
		___
		434

Step 2:	Total manhours for the same period.	1,398,765
		1,456,732
		1,129,565
		1,623,451
		1,834,225
		_____
		7,442,738

Step 3: Apply the formula and compute the cumulative accident rate.

$$Rate = \frac{H \& I \; Recordables \times 200,000}{Total \; hours \; worked}$$

$$Rate = \frac{434 \times 200,000}{7,442,743}$$

$$Rate = \frac{86,800,000}{7,442,743}$$

$$Rate = 11.7$$

83) We selected answer D because:

There are many formats for lesson plans. However, the most widely used format includes the following areas:

Title: Indicates subject matter being taught. Should be clear and concise.

Objectives: Should indicate the purpose of the session or goals. Specifically, it should indicate what the students are

	expected to know or be able to do at the end of the session or lesson.
Aids:	A list of all training aids such as videos, equipment, charts, etc. to be used to develop important points in the lesson.
Introduction:	Every lesson should be introduced to the class in a manner that will develop the interest of the group. It should give the students the scope and importance of the subject.
Presentation:	This is the plan of action. It is the guide for putting across the ideas, information or skills the student should learn. It should indicate the method of presentation ie; lecture, demonstration, guided discussion etc.
Application:	If possible application examples should be illustrated either by student experience or by an illustration by the instructor.
Summary:	The summary restates the main points of the lesson and helps to strengthen the weak points in the instruction.

84) We selected answer C because:

The three most often recommended fundamental training courses for general industrial workers are: First Aid, Fire Extinguisher, and Contingency. Contingency meaning emergency procedures.

85) We selected answer A because:

Obviously, no safety poster can substitute for the active and sincere interest of the company management.

86) We selected answer A because:

Supervisors are in the best position to provide realistic and effective training for industrial workers. They have detailed knowledge of work processes and control workflow.

87) We selected answer A because:

Incidence rate is the rate of development of *"new cases"* of a specific disease over a given time period.

88) We selected answer B because:

Brainstorming is a technique of group interactions that encourages each participant to present ideas on a specific issue. The method is normally used to find new, innovative approaches to issues. There are four ground rules:

- Ideas presented are not criticized.
- Freewheeling creative thinking and building on ideas are positively reinforced.
- As many ideas as possible should be presented quickly.
- Combining several ideas or improving suggestions is encouraged.

89) We selected answer A because:

Role playing is ideally suited for human relations education or training. It allows the students to become participants in a "drama" or "play" that depicts the interaction of humans during stressful or error provocative situations. The technique is not suited for problem solving or technical training.

90) We selected answer D because:

The OSHA DART is useful in industrial safety work as an indicator of an accident frequency rate to compare your organization's accident severity and frequency against other similar industry rates.

91) We selected answer C because:

The Ground-Fault Circuit Interrupter is a fast-action device, which senses a small current leakage to ground and, in a fraction of a second, shuts off the electricity and *interrupts* the faulty flow to ground. Placed between the electrical service and the tool or appliance it serves, the GFCI continually matches the amount of current going to and from the tool along the normal path of the circuit conductors. Whenever the amount *going* differs from the amount *returning* by a set trip level the GFCI interrupts the electric power within 1/40th of a second. This difference in current is called leakage current to ground and the path it takes to ground could be through a person - in which case, the rapid response of the GFCI is fast enough to prevent electrocution. This protection provided by the GFCI is independent of the condition of the equipment grounding conductor, thus, the GFCI can provide protection even if the equipment grounding conductor becomes inoperative. **The device will not detect line-to-line faults.**

92) We selected answer A because:

Per the OSHA code firewalls separating fuel and oxygen cylinders must have at least a 30 minute rating and be at least 5 feet high. This is discussed in OSHA 1910.252.

93) We selected answer D because:

In accordance with OSHA 1910.147 (c)(4)(ii) individual energy control procedures are required for machines or equipment that have more than one energy source, that is, they must be locked out at different locations to ensure safety. These individual procedures must contain provisions for outlining the techniques to be used for each machine. They must include:

- specific steps for shutting down the machine
- specific steps for the placement, removal and transfer of lockout or tagout devices
- specific steps to test the machine or equipment to ensure the isolation of energy

94) We selected answer D because:

The National Fire Protection Association publishes the Fire Protection Handbook.

95) We selected answer D because:

The person to correct the hazard should be the individual with the most knowledge of the area that is the area supervisor.

96) We selected answer D because:

This can be a difficult question, but the BEST answer of those listed it to only make recommendations based on your competencies if you are sure that the result will ensure a safer work area. Making recommendations about areas that you are not knowledgeable in has the potential to be incorrect.

97) We selected answer C because:

CM rules are outlined in the Certification Maintenance Guide and it states:

"A failure to meet your continuous maintenance (CM) requirements results in your OHST or CHST certification being revoked. You may re-acquire the certification by paying the examination fee (reapplication is not required) and passing the current OHST or CHST examination. You must complete this activity within five years of being notified that the certification is no longer valid.

If more than five years passes after losing your OHST or CHST certification because CM requirements were not met, you must seek the certification as a new applicant."

98) We selected answer A because:

The first action should be to contact the supervisor who has control of the workplace and discuss the infraction. Further action may include some of the other solutions presented in the above options.

99) We selected answer B because:

The GHS Working Group identified about 35 different types of information that are currently required on labels by different systems. To harmonize, key information elements needed to be identified. Additional harmonization may occur on other elements in time, in particular for precautionary statements. The elements identified below are
*Standardized:

> Product identifier
> Supplier identifier
> Chemical identity
> Hazard pictograms*
> Signal words*
> Hazard statements*
> Precautionary information

100) Answer C is correct because:

Chemical Resistant Glove

- *Butyl*: High resistance protection from gas or water vapors. Also, resistant to common acids and alcohols.
- *Hot-Mill or Aluminized Glove*: Reflective and insulating protection, for welding, furnace and foundry work.
- *Latex*: Protection from most aqueous solutions of acids, alkalis, salts and ketones. They resist abrasions during grinding, sandblasting and polishing. These general-purpose, pliable and comfortable gloves are used for common industrial applications, food processing, maintenance, construction and lab work.
- *Natural Rubber*: Liquid-proof protection against acids, caustics and dye stuffs.
- *Neoprene*: Protection against hydraulic fluids, gasoline, alcohols, organic acids and alkalis. They offer good pliability and finger dexterity, high density, tensile strength, plus high tear resistance.
- *Neoprene Latex*: Protection against detergents, salts, acids and caustic solutions.
- *Nitrile/Natural Rubber*: Protection from chlorinated solvents. They are intended for jobs requiring dexterity and sensitivity. Nitrile/Rubber blend resists abrasions, cuts, tears

and punctures.

- *N-DEX Glove*: These nitrile gloves provide splash and spill protection against a wide variety of chemicals, although not intended for extended immersion activities. Available in low-power and powder-free options.
- *Polyvinyl Alcohol (PVA) Glove*: Resistance to strong solvents such as chlorinated and aromatic solvents. This material is water soluble (polyvinyl alcohol) and cannot be used in water or water-based solutions.
- *Polyvinyl Chloride (PVC) Glove*: Resistance to abrasives such as materials coated or immersed in grease, oil, acids or caustics. Available lined or unlined depending on dexterity requirements.
- *Silver Shield Glove*: Protection against a wide range of solvents, acids and bases. This lightweight laminate is flexible, but not form-fitting, which affects user dexterity.
- *Vinyl Glove*: Resistance to a variety of irritants.
- *Viton Glove*: Resistance to PCBs, chlorinated and aromatic solvents, gas and water vapors. These gloves can be used in water-based solutions.

Self-Assessment Exam Two Questions

1) Which of the elements listed below belong to the halogen group?
   A) Na, Ca, K.
   B) C, O, H.
   C) F, Cl, Br, I.
   D) Au, Ag, Pt.

2) The pneumoconiosis that is caused by inhalation of iron oxide is called?
   A) Anthracosis.
   B) Siderosis.
   C) Silicosis.
   D) Silicosiderosis.

3) If a vessel contains 80% air and 20% hydrocarbons, what is the oxygen content of the vessel?
   A) 14%
   B) 21%
   C) 16.8%
   D) 15.5%

4) The tool rest on a grinding wheel should be _____ away from the wheel.
   A) 1/4 inch.
   B) 1/2 inch.
   C) 1/3 inch.
   D) 1 inch.

5) An elevator daily spot check should include which of the following?
   A) V-Groove.
   B) Governor.
   C) Cable gripper jaws.
   D) Brakes.

6) Which of the following measurements does the inverse square law **not** apply to?
   A) Heat.
   B) Illumination.
   C) Noise.
   D) Radiation.

7) Damage to the eyes of an unprotected observer from the flash of an
    electric welder's arc could be caused by the exposure to:
    A) Infrared light.
    B) Invisible radiation.
    C) Ultraviolet radiation.
    D) Sensible light.

8) When conducting a fire investigation, the number one area to be
    determined is?
    A) Fire ignition sequence.
    B) Response time.
    C) Number of deaths.
    D) Were all building and fire codes followed in construction.

9) Carbon tetrachloride is **most likely** to cause damage to the _____.
    A) Heart.
    B) Lungs.
    C) Liver.
    D) Bones.

10) In the design of a ventilation system, which of the following operations
    would require the greatest capture velocity?
    A) Evaporation from open surface tanks.
    B) Spray booths.
    C) Welding.
    D) Grinding.

11) What is the desired air velocity (fpm) at relief or spot cooling stations for
    activity that produces extremely high heat loads for workers?
    A) 50 fpm.
    B) 100 fpm.
    C) 125 fpm.
    D) 4000 fpm.

12) Using the formula (N-18) x 5 rem, what is the long-term radiation
    accumulation permitted for a 49 year old reactor worker?
    A) 125 rem.
    B) 155 rem.
    C) 255 rem.
    D) 15,000 mr.

13) The ability to accurately read a color-change detector tube or badge depends to a large extent on the ability of the observer and the lighting conditions. Which of the following conditions provides the **best** opportunity for obtaining a precise reading of colorimetric tubes?
    A)   Fluorescent lighting of at least 150 foot candles.
    B)   Daylight or incandescent lighting.
    C)   Mercury vapor lighting.
    D)   A 10,000 watt sun gun .

14) A welding operator using argon for shielding gas would **most likely** be welding which of the following materials?
    A)   Tungsten.
    B)   Galvanized Steel.
    C)   Copper.
    D)   Aluminum.

15) In statistical development, which of the following terms would indicate the amount of dispersion in a frequency distribution?
    A)   Mode & Median.
    B)   Range and Standard Deviation.
    C)   Standard Deviation and Mean.
    D)   Mean, Range and Standard Deviation.

16) A storage tank contains residual pooled toluene, which has a vapor pressure of 28 mm Hg. What is the maximum concentration of toluene vapor within the tank?
    A)   12%
    B)   3.7%
    C)   6.7%
    D)   21.3%

17) Exposure to coal tar products has been shown to increase the adverse effects from which of the following?
    A)   Chromates.
    B)   Acetone.
    C)   UV Radiation.
    D)   IR Radiation.

18) Which of the following is the correct title for the accident prevention manual published by the Factory Mutual system?
   A) Handbook of Industrial Loss Prevention.
   B) Manual of Occupational Safety.
   C) Occupational Safety Handbook.
   D) Industrial Safety Engineering Manual.

19) Which of the following is the **best** description of a Mist?
   A) Suspension of liquid particles in air.
   B) Suspension of liquid or solid particles in air.
   C) Solid particle in air formed by condensation.
   D) Particulate material in air.

20) When using a solid sorbent tube for personal sampling which of the following would be considered the **most important?**
   A) Place the tube in the breathing zone.
   B) Spike blanks to check the laboratory QC.
   C) Ship bulk samples in a separate package.
   D) Use plastic caps instead of tape to seal tube at end of sampling.

21) A KV factor indicates the strokes per cc of air drawn through a hand operated sampling pump. What would the factor be for 960 pumps and 0.75 liters of air?
   A) 1.28
   B) 10.28
   C) .78
   D) 78

22) Which of the following elements is a stronger oxidizer than oxygen?
   A) Fluorine.
   B) Chlorine.
   C) Bromine.
   D) Sulfuric acid.

23) Calculate the WBGT index from the following information, an indoor globe temperature of 91°F and a wet-bulb temperature of 87°F.
  A) 112.2°F
  B) 92°F
  C) 88.2°F
  D) 34°C

24) Why is rectal temperature used in heat stress evaluation?
  A) Indicates true temperature.
  B) Much more accurate than oral temperature.
  C) Indicates "core" body temperature.
  D) An old standard that has never been changed.

25) Which of the following **best** describes the greatest single error in colorimetric sampling devices?
  A) Gel coagulation.
  B) Temperature extremes.
  C) Pump airflow inaccuracy.
  D) Interferences by other contaminants.

26) According to 29 CFR 1910.23, a standard railing shall consist of top rail, intermediate rail, and posts, and shall have a vertical height of ___ inches nominal from upper surface of top rail to floor, platform, runway, or ramp level.
  A) 36.
  B) 40.
  C) 42.
  D) 48.

27) A radioisotope has a half-life of 1 year. How many years will it take to reduce the initial activity to less than 10%?
  A) 1 year.
  B) 2 years.
  C) 3 years.
  D) 4 years.

28) When discussing the cleaning of plant air in a ventilation system the process that uses carbon to remove contaminants or undesirable odors is known as:
   A) Adsorption.
   B) Absorption.
   C) Combustion.
   D) Condensation.

29) Which of the following correctly indicates the amount of contaminant remaining in a vessel after a purge of 5 volumes?

   $$C = C_o \ e^{-w/v}$$

   A) About 7%
   B) About 10%
   C) 0.67%
   D) 67%

   WHERE C = Final Concentration
   C_o = Initial Concentration
   w = Withdrawn Volume
   v = Volume

30) What is the velocity in feet per minute in a duct with a flanged round opening if the hood static pressure is 2.45 in. water and the coefficient of entry is 0.82?
   A) 8675 fpm.
   B) 5140 fpm.
   C) 4460 fpm.
   D) 9000 fpm.

31) The chance of a dust cloud igniting is governed by what?
   A) Oxygen content and dust accumulation.
   B) Size of dust particles and impurities present.
   C) Strength of the source of ignition.
   D) All of the responses listed.

32) A 6 inch diameter grinding wheel rotating at 500 rpm has a surface speed of?
   A) 556 ft/min.
   B) 690 ft/min.
   C) 785 ft/min.
   D) 9425 ft/min.

33) If 3500 cfm of air is drawn through an 8-inch diameter duct, what is the velocity in feet per minute?
   A) 1023 fpm.
   B) 10,230 fpm.
   C) 800 fpm.
   D) 1000 fpm.

$$Q = A\ V$$

34) Given a velocity pressure reading of 0.60 in a circular duct, what is the velocity in feet per minute?
   A) 3102 fpm.
   B) 15 fpm.
   C) 29 fpm.
   D) 1023 m

$$V = 4005\sqrt{.60}$$

35) Compute the TWA concentration for the following measurements: 0800-0900 hrs. @ 400ppm--0900-1100 hrs. @ 600ppm--1100-1300 hrs. @ 10ppm---1300-1400 hrs. @ 100---1400-1600 hrs. @ 300.
   A) 200 ppm.
   B) 133 ppm.
   C) 113 ppm.
   D) 290 ppm.

36) Based on the allowable limits in the table below, if the noise in a work area was 95 dBA for 3 hrs, 90 dBA for 4 hrs and 85 dBA for 2 hrs, is the allowable limit exceeded?
   A) Yes, by about 25%.
   B) No, but almost.
   C) No, less than half.
   D) Yes, by almost double.

PERMISSIBLE NOISE EXPOSURES					
Hrs	dBA	Hrs	dBA	Hrs	dBA
8	90	3	97	1	105
6	92	2	100	0.5	110
4	95	1.5	102	0.25	115

37) A test atmosphere is prepared using 2.5 mL of pure CO in a 190 L container. What is the concentration of CO?
   A) 132 ppm.
   B) 13 ppm.
   C) 22 ppm.
   D) 88 ppm.

38) A pump was calibrated at a flow rate of 1.8 L/min while connected to a representative sampler. A sample was taken in the field for 4 hours and 20 minutes. The filter starting weight was 0.003422 gram and the after sampling weight was 0.004442 gram. What is the concentration in mg/m^3?
   A) 1.96 mg/m^3.
   B) 1.02 mg/m^3.
   C) 2.18 mg/m^3.
   D) 3.47 mg/m^3.

39) The pressure inside a sealed drum is 12.5 Psi at 55 degrees F. when it leaves the loading dock in California. What is the pressure inside the drum when it reaches Nevada and the temperature is 120 degrees F? Assume the temperature inside the sealed drum has stabilized at 120 degrees F.
   A) 27.3 Psi.
   B) 16.0 Psi.
   C) 14 Psi.
   D) Volume of drum must be known.

40) Which of the following does **not** require an equipment grounding conductor?
   A) A double reverse delta electrical system.
   B) A double insulated hand tool.
   C) A circuit that is protected with circuit breakers.
   D) A system with a wye connected transformer.

41) Authorized Powered Industrial Truck drivers must be re-evaluated once every:
   A) Year.
   B) 6 Months.
   C) 2 Years.
   D) 3 Years.

42) Which one of the following system safety tools would **not** be appropriate for analysis of a complex system?
    A)   Fault Tree Analysis.
    B)   Multilinear Events Sequencing.
    C)   Job Safety Analysis.
    D)   Failure Modes and Effect Analysis.

43) Which of the following agencies is the **best** source for standards dealing with the adequacy and placement of fire extinguishers?
    A)   ANSI.
    B)   NFPA.
    C)   MSHA.
    D)   EPA.

44) All of the following are active environmental, health or safety laws **except?**
    A)   Clean Air Act.
    B)   National Environmental Policy Act.
    C)   Safe Drinking Water Act.
    D)   Hazardous Transportation Act.

45) Which of the following acts was enacted first?
    A)   Federal Coal Mine Health and Safety Act.
    B)   The Occupational Health and Safety Act.
    C)   The Toxic Substance Control Act.
    D)   The Metal and Non-metallic Mine Safety Act.

46) A truck carrying chemicals has been involved in an accident. The only information about the materials on board is that the pH is 1.5. What does this tell you about the toxicity of the cargo?
    A)   Cargo has a flash point below 100 degrees F.
    B)   Cargo has a flash point above 100 degrees F.
    C)   Cargo is an acid.
    D)   Cargo is a base.

47) Which of the following is **not** a valid RCRA characteristic of hazardous waste?
   A) Ignitability.
   B) Corrosivity.
   C) Reactivity.
   D) Radioactivity.

48) According to 40 CFR, generators of hazardous waste must develop all of the following **except?**
   A) A written inspection plan.
   B) A written contingency plan.
   C) A written waste analysis plan.
   D) Fire and emergency services onsite.

49) Which of the following firefighting agents could be effectively used on a Class "A" fire?
   A) Purple K.
   B) Halon 1301.
   C) Dry Chemical (Potassium Chloride).
   D) Dry Chemical (Ammonium Phosphate).

50) A worker at your plant was overcome in a confined space. Another worker who was sent to rescue him was also overcome. Which one of the following types of respiratory protective equipment is the **best** choice for the next rescuer?
   A) Air Line Respirator with chemical cartridge escape.
   B) Gas Mask.
   C) Air Supplied Hood with escape bottle.
   D) Self Contained Breathing Apparatus.

51) You are responding to a confined space where one person has entered and is now presumed dead. Which of the following instruments would you take with you?
   A) CGI with Oxygen sensor.
   B) IR Spectrometer.
   C) GCMS.
   D) Pitot Tube.

52) A truck carrying chemicals for your plant has just been involved in an accident. The only information the first responders can provide you is that the materials on board have a pH of 9.0. What does this tell you about the toxicity of the cargo?
    A) Cargo has a flash point below 100 degrees F.
    B) Cargo has a flash point above 100 degrees F.
    C) Cargo is an acid.
    D) Cargo is a base.

53) According to 29 CFR 1910.120, newly assigned personnel that are assigned as First Responders, but have not been training may:
    A) Not respond.
    B) Respond only in a real emergency.
    C) Respond only under the supervision of a trained responder.
    D) May be a responder if trained within the first 90 days of being assigned to the position.

54) Once a chemical has been classified, the hazard(s) must be communicated to target audiences. The exhibited pictogram represents which hazard class?
    A) Carcinogen.
    B) Irritant.
    C) Acute toxicity.
    D) Environmental Toxicity

55) The Science of Ergonomics deals with all of the following **except?**
    A) Anthropometry.
    B) Automation.
    C) Autokinesis.
    D) Autotrophic.

56) Phosgene (COCl2) contains what proportion by weight of chlorine?
    A) 50%
    B) 60%
    C) 70%
    D) 35%

*Note: Molecular weight of C = 12, Oxygen = 16, Chlorine = 35.5.

57) Although the use of the term torr has been discouraged the term is still used quite often. Torr is a unit of high vacuum and is equal to?
   A) One inch of water column.
   B) 29.92 inches of mercury.
   C) One mm of mercury.
   D) One inch of lead.

58) Which of the following chemical equations is balanced?
   PbS + 2HCl ⟶

   A) PbCl2 + H2S.
   B) Pb2 + H4O4.
   C) H2S4.
   D) 4PbS(HCl).

59) A motorcycle is traveling at 45 mph. If the driver's reaction time is .75 seconds, how many meters will the vehicle travel between the time the driver sees a problem and actually applies the brakes?
   A) 15 meters.
   B) 25 meters.
   C) 18 meters.
   D) 50 meters.

60) In developing a safety training program, the **most essential** consideration is:
   A) Training staff.
   B) Training methods.
   C) Content of training program.
   D) Training objectives.

61) Which of the following laws states: Pressure times Volume = a constant number?
   A) Charles' law.
   B) Watts' law.
   C) Newton's law.
   D) Boyle's law.

62) One Curie = 3.7 x 1010 disintegrations per second. One Curie is equal to how many disintegrations per minute?
    A)   6.2 x 108.
    B)   6.2 x 1012.
    C)   2.22 x 1012.
    D)   2.22 x 108.

63) If X + Y = 9 and 3X - 2Y = 7, then X = _____ and Y = _____.
    A)   X = 4 and Y = 5.
    B)   X = 5 and Y = 4.
    C)   X = 7 and Y = 2.
    D)   X = 3 and Y = 6.

64) The Celsius scale is the same as the Centigrade temperature scale.
    A)   True.
    B)   False.

65) If 5X - 7 = 3X - 3, then what is the value of X?
    A)   4.
    B)   5.
    C)   2.
    D)   3.

66) A temperature of 70 degrees C equals _____ degrees Kelvin.
    A)   273.
    B)   373.
    C)   203.
    D)   343.

67) Which widely circulated loss control and insurance **best** describes the types of losses that various industries face?
    A)   Best's Loss Control Engineering Manual.
    B)   The Grey House Safety & Security Directory.
    C)   OSHA 29 CFR 1910.
    D)   Robert's Industry Loss Manual.

68) How many carbon atoms does a benzene ring have?
   A) 4.
   B) 5.
   C) 6.
   D) 8.

69) What is the **primary** recommended use for a canopy hood?
   A) Welding.
   B) Hot processes.
   C) Paint spray booth.
   D) Degreasing tanks.

70) Which of the following conversions is **not** correct?
   A) $1 ft^3 = 7.48$ gallons.
   B) $1 m^3 = 100$ Liters.
   C) 1 gal = 128 oz.
   D) 1 gal = 3.79 Liters.

71) Which of the following is **most correct** concerning the safety afforded by building codes?
   A) Building codes ensure safety of all concerned.
   B) Building codes should be considered paramount.
   C) Codes protect construction workers.
   D) Codes represent the minimum requirements for materials and construction.

72) When supplying breathing air to five or more abrasive blasting respirators, what is the minimum amount of air to be supplied to each unit?
   A) 3 CFM.
   B) 6 CFM.
   C) 9 CFM.
   D) 12 CFM.

73) Which of the following ANSI Standards deal with elevators?
   A) ANSI Z16.1
   B) ANSI A17.1
   C) ANSI Z87.1
   D) ANSI Z89.1

74) All of the following actions are required of a company that receives an OSHA citation **except?**
    A) Pay the fine.
    B) Pay the fine and post the notice of violation.
    C) Correct the violation.
    D) Retrain all employees.

75) The ANSI standard that covers construction Hard Hats is?
    A) ANSI Z87.1
    B) ANSI B16.4
    C) ANSI A12.1
    D) ANSI Z89.1

76) Which of the following Code of Federal Regulations (CFR) deals with Protection of the Environment?
    A) 10 CFR.
    B) 20 CFR.
    C) 40 CFR.
    D) 42 CFR.

77) Which of the following precautions would be the **least effective** against occupational dermatoses?
    A) Frequent washing of the face and hands with an organic solvent followed by soap and water.
    B) Use of good housekeeping and frequent washing with soap and water.
    C) Good hygiene practices and use of gloves.
    D) Frequent washing with soap and water and the use of barrier cream.

78) A gas mask is to be used for protection against Carbon Monoxide. What color should the canister be?
    A) Blue.
    B) Black.
    C) Yellow.
    D) Green.

79) Which of the following techniques would be the preferred control method for preventing exposure to a hazardous noise exposure?
    A) Control employee work hours to reduce exposure time.
    B) Engineer a less hazardous environment.
    C) Provide protective equipment.
    D) Automate the process to reduce worker interaction.

80) Based on a qualitative fit test, what is the protection factor afforded by a half-mask face piece respirator?
    A) 1.
    B) 10.
    C) 100.
    D) 1000.

81) Grab samples are used for?
    A) 8-hour average.
    B) Never used.
    C) To identify peak or ceiling concentration.
    D) To calculate a TWA for the work shift.

82) Which of the following is an unacceptable method of protecting an employee from a radiant heat source?
    A) Reducing the temperature of the infrared source.
    B) Provide infrared shadows.
    C) Reflecting protective equipment.
    D) Increase ventilation.

83) In industrial environments the concept of local exhaust ventilation is used extensively. The purpose of local exhaust ventilation is to:
    A) Prevent any entrance of air contaminants.
    B) Remove contaminants at their source.
    C) Provide dilution ventilation.
    D) Provide spot ventilation for comfort.

84) Which of the following concerning dilution ventilation is correct? Dilution ventilation is used to:
    A) Control a contaminant at its source.
    B) Control fumes from lead fusing.
    C) Control low toxicity vapors.
    D) Control asbestos fibers.

85) Given equal thicknesses, which substance would be the **most effective** shield for gamma rays?
   A) Cement.
   B) Water.
   C) Sheet Steel.
   D) Lead.

86) Which of the following is **not** a requirement for a flammable liquid "Safety" can?
   A) Spring loaded cover that opens at 5 psi.
   B) Flame arrestor.
   C) Fusible link.
   D) Metal construction.

87) During qualitative fit testing, which of the following are the test subjects required to read?
   A) A newspaper article about respirators use.
   B) The Gettysburg Address.
   C) The Rainbow Passage.
   D) The Safety Motto.

88) General or dilution ventilation is appropriate in all of the following **except?**
   A) When small quantities of contaminants are released.
   B) The toxicity of contaminants is low.
   C) Air is not drawn through the workers' breathing zone.
   D) Corrosion may occur to equipment in the workroom.

89) Which of the following terms is used to indicate the volume of air inhaled and exhaled in a normal human breath?
   A) Residual volume.
   B) Tidal volume.
   C) Supplemental air.
   D) Vital capacity.

90) All of the following are disadvantages of fabric collectors **except?**
   A) Can be a fire or explosive hazard.
   B) Some fabric materials may be hard to clean.
   C) Does not work well with moist gas.
   D) Has very poor efficiency.

91) During the starting sequence of a gas fired drying oven any accumulation of flammable gases should be reduced to _____% of the Lower Flammable Limit?
   A) 0%
   B) 5%
   C) 15%
   D) 25%

92) When is the use of a Gas Mask permissible in an atmosphere that is Immediately Dangerous to Life or Health due to the presence of a toxic contaminant?
   A) Never.
   B) When it is used for escape only.
   C) As a backup measure.
   D) When SCBA is being inspected.

93) Which of the following would **most likely** result in the immediate functioning of an electrical magnetic circuit breaker to interrupt the current?
   A) Undersize wiring.
   B) A line-to-line short.
   C) A 20% overload for any period of time.
   D) Ground fault.

94) Which of the following **best** describes the function of barrier cream?
   A) Replaces lanolin in the skin.
   B) Keeps hands clean.
   C) Inhibits contact of solvent with skin surface.
   D) A cure for chapped, dry hands and feet.

95) In which case could a double-insulated, two-wire portable drill, produce a shock hazard?
   A)   All cases, it requires a third ground wire.
   B)   Short between white and black wire.
   C)   Short between case and black wire.
   D)   If the energized drill was dropped in water.

96) Carpal tunnel syndrome is a repetitive motion disease that affects many production workers. Recently efforts to prevent injuries in the red meat industry have met with great success. The symptoms of Carpal tunnel syndrome include all of the following **except?**
   A)   Numbness in little finger.
   B)   Pain in the wrist upon exertion.
   C)   Pain in the second and third fingers.
   D)   Inflammation and swelling of the wrist.

97) Damage to the eyes of an unprotected observer from the flash of an electric welder's arc could be caused by the exposure to:
   A)   Infrared light.
   B)   Invisible radiation.
   C)   Ultraviolet radiation.
   D)   Sensible light.

98) What is the **primary** reason for safety training? Choose the best answer.
   A)   Improve skills.
   B)   Behavior change.
   C)   Keep the training department busy.
   D)   Comply with federal law.

99) One of the **most important** steps in the establishment of a training program is to set sound, obtainable objectives. In which part of the training program development should objectives be established?
   A)   As early as possible.
   B)   Toward the end of development.
   C)   Before equipment money is allocated.
   D)   When instructors are hired.

100) The physiological property of matter that defines the capacity of a chemical to harm or injure a living organism by other than mechanical means is the definition for?
    A)   Illness.
    B)   Toxicity.
    C)   Injury.
    D)   Pollution.

Self-Assessment Exam Two Answers

1) We selected answer C because:

The halogen group consists of these elements: Fluorine, Chlorine, Bromine, and Iodine.

2) We selected answer B because:

Anthracosis is a pneumoconiosis caused by the exposure to coal dust (black lung). *Silicosis* is a pneumoconiosis caused by inhalation of the dust of stone, sand, or flint containing silica. **Siderosis** is a lung disease caused by inhalation of iron oxide or other metallic particles. *Silicosiderosis* is a pneumoconiosis in which the inhaled dust is that of silica and iron.

3) We selected answer C because:

Normal air contains 21% oxygen by volume. The question states: the vessel only contains 80% normal air. Therefore:

$$0.21 \times .80 = 0.168 = 16.8\%$$

4) We selected answer A because:

Of the choices offered - always keep the tool rest 1/4 inch from the working edge of the wheel is the best answer. However, you will find 1/8 inch as the required distance in most safety literature. As a test strategy, I would answer 1/8 of an inch if that is an option, however if 1/4 is the lowest number, then select it.

5) We selected answer D because:

According to the NSC Accident Prevention Manual (Administration and Programs) daily spot checks of elevators should be conducted at the beginning of each day and include: level floor stops, testing of the alarm bell, brakes, and other mechanical operations. Selection A "V-Groove" refers to older friction equipment in which the hoisting rope is not attached to the machine. The elevator is moved by the traction of the ropes in v-groves on the drive pulley. The V-groove would require monthly inspection. Selection B "Governor" refers to a speed control device that is normally checked monthly. Selection C "Cable gripper jaws" refers to cable grabbing devices that hold governors, counter weights or the car itself, which are inspected annually.

6) We selected answer A because:

You can use the inverse square law for measurements concerning noise, illumination and radiation but not heat.

7) We selected answer C because:

Damage to the eyes from ultraviolet radiation is much more violent than those of the visible or infrared, a severe burn can be produced with little or no warning and significant damage to the lens of the eye can occur.

8) We selected answer A because:

To determine the root cause, you need to determine the fire ignition source and the area of origin.

9) We selected answer C because:

Carbon tetrachloride (Carbon Tet) is an outlawed solvent that causes damage to the liver.

10) We selected answer D because:

Grinding operations create large amounts of contaminants at very high initial velocities, thus demanding higher capture velocities to secure the contaminates. All of the other operations listed generate contaminants with low velocities.

11) We selected answer D because:

The amount of air motion acceptable to a worker performing extremely heavy work at relief stations would be in the vicinity of 3000 to 4000 fpm. Moderate loads would require about 2000 to 3000 fpm and light loads about 1000 to 2000. Ref. ACGIH Industrial Ventilation Manual.

12) We selected answer B because:

$$(N - 18) \times 5 \text{ rem}$$

$$(49 - 18) \times 5 \text{ rem}$$

$$(31) \times 5 = 155 \text{ rem}$$

13) We selected answer B because:

Exposed detectors should be examined in bright sunlight or with incandescent lighting. Mercury vapor lighting sometimes makes it difficult to observe color change. Fluorescent lighting should also be avoided because they do not provide a good match for some colors.

14) We selected answer D because:

The two most common shielded gas welding processes are MIG (Metallic Inert Gas Welding) & TIG (Tungsten Inert Gas). The process is used on Aluminum with a shielding gas of argon or helium. Carbon dioxide would be used as a shield if the process was to be used on steel.

15) We selected answer B because:

The *Range* is a measure of variability or difference between the highest and lowest values in a frequency distribution. The *Standard Deviation* is an average of all the measurements of deviation from the mean in a sample or random variable. The Range and Standard Deviation are both measures of dispersion of a frequency distribution.

16)   We selected answer B because:

$$\frac{28}{760} = 0.036842 = 3.7\%$$

17)   We selected answer C because:

Exposure to the Ultraviolet Radiation from the sun in combination with exposure to coal tar products has resulted in a significant number of workers experiencing a photosensitization of the skin.

18)   We selected answer A because:

The correct title for the FM accident prevention manual is the "Handbook of Industrial Loss Prevention".

19)   We selected answer A because:

Historically there have been questions on the examination concerning the definition of the following.

- Mist - Suspension of liquid particles in air formed by condensation from vapor or by some mechanical process (40 - 400μm)
- Aerosol - Suspension of liquid or solid particles in air
- Dust - Particulate material generated by a mechanical process (0.5 - 50 μm)
- Fume - Solid particle aerosol formed by condensation from the vapor state (0.001 - 0.2μm)
- Smoke - aerosol formed from combustion of organic material (0.01 - 0.5μm)

20) We selected answer A because:

Although all of the other selections are very important in ensuring an accurate and dependable sampling, placement of the tube in the breathing zone is a primary consideration.

21) We selected answer A because:

$$KV = \frac{strokes}{cc}$$

$$KV = \frac{960}{750}$$

$$KV = 1.28$$

*Note: $1cc = 1cm^3 = 1ml$

22) We selected answer A because:

All of the listed materials are oxidizers, however the only element stronger than oxygen is *fluorine*!

23) We selected answer C because:

$$WBGT = 0.7\,WB + 0.3\,GT$$

$$WBGT = (0.7 \times 87) + (0.3 \times 91)$$

$$WBGT = 60.9 + 27.3$$

$$WBGT = 88.2^{\circ}\,F$$

24) We selected answer C because:

The rectal temperature is normally used in evaluations of heat stress because it indicates "core" temperature and is not subject to the fluctuations associated with oral temperature. Oral temperature may rise or fall depending on respiration rate, relative humidity, type of breathing and many other factors. Normally a temperature rise of up to 1° C is allowed.

25) We selected answer D because:

Although all the other answers are factors when using colorimetric sampling devices, interferences by other contaminants is by far the largest single error factor when using these samplers.

26) We selected answer C because:

29 CFR 1910.23(e)(1): A standard railing shall consist of top rail, intermediate rail, and posts, and shall have a vertical height of 42 inches nominal from upper surface of top rail to floor, platform, runway, or ramp level. The top rail shall be smooth-surfaced throughout the length of the railing. The intermediate rail shall be approximately halfway between the top rail and the floor, platform, runway, or ramp. The ends of the rails shall not overhang the terminal posts except where such overhang does not constitute a projection hazard.

29 CFR 1910.23(e)(4): A standard toeboard shall be 4 inches nominal in vertical height from its top edge to the level of the floor, platform, runway, or ramp. It shall be securely fastened in place and with not more than 1/4-inch clearance above floor level. It may be made of any substantial material either solid or with openings not over 1 inch in greatest dimension.

27) We selected answer D because:

The activity after three years will be 12.5% of the initial activity. After 4 years, the activity will be 6.25% of the initial activity.

$$100\% \quad 1^{st}\ yr \quad = 50\%$$
$$50\% \quad 2^{nd}\ yr \quad = 25\%$$
$$25\% \quad 3^{rd}\ yr \quad = 12.5\%$$
$$12.5\% \quad 4^{th}\ yr \quad = 6.25\%$$

28) We selected answer A because:

All of the processes listed are used in air cleaning of gases and vapors. However the method cited is that of *Adsorption*. Adsorption involves an action that takes place at the surface of the adsorbent material where gas and solid make contact. The most widely used adsorbent for cleaning air is activated carbon, which most often is placed in canisters, perforated cans or trays. Activated carbon has the ability to adsorb gases and vapors up to about 60% of its own weight. If the carbon is then heated the captured material can then be reclaimed, making it an attractive and cost effective process. *Condensation* is the process of lowering the temperature of the incoming air to change the vapor to a liquid state. The process uses various chillers, condensers or refrigeration units to lower the temperature of the vapor. *Combustion* is a process used for removal of gas or vapor if it can be oxidized to a harmless or odor free state. Many times this takes the form of a direct-flame afterburner. Catalysts are also used to great effect in paint disposal, animal fats, plastics etc. *Absorption* is the process of using a liquid, which dissolves or chemically reacts with the gas or vapor that is to be removed.

29) We selected answer C because:

$$C = C_o\ e^{-w/v}$$

$$C = 1.0 \times 2.71828^{-5/1}$$

$$C = 0.00673$$

$$C = 0.00673 \times 100\% = 0.673\%$$

30) We selected answer B because:

$$V = 4005 \ C_e \ \sqrt{SP_h}$$

$$V = 4005 \times 0.82 \times \sqrt{2.45 \ in.water}$$

$$V = 4005 \times 0.82 \times 1.565$$

$$V = 5140 \ fpm$$

31) We selected answer D because:

All of these factors govern the possibility of a dust explosion. Dust explosions usually occur as a series, the initial deflagration being rather small in volume but intense enough to jar dust from beams, ledges, etc. This causes larger concentrations to form and a second more destructive cycle will begin.

32) We selected answer C because:

$$C = \pi \times d$$

$$C = (3.14) \times \left(\tfrac{6}{12} \ ft\right) = 1.57 \ ft$$

$$SFM = C \times RPM$$

$$SFM = 1.57 \ ft/R \times 500 \ RPM = 785 \ ft \ per \ min$$

*Note: The conversion from 6 inches to 0.5 feet early in the process is a time saver and simplifies the conversion process (small numbers rather than large numbers). One valuable technique is to check the answers after reading the question to see what units are required. Then you can do your conversion up front, if beneficial.

33)   We selected answer B because:

$$Q = A \; V$$

$$V = \frac{Q}{A}$$

$$A = \pi \, r^2$$

$$A = 3.14 \times \left(\tfrac{4}{12} \; ft\right)^2$$

$$V = \frac{3500}{0.342}$$

$$V = 10{,}230 \; fpm$$

34)   We selected answer A because:

$$V = 4005 \sqrt{.60}$$

$$V = 4005 \times .77459$$

$$V = 3102 \; fpm$$

35) We selected answer D because:

$$TWA = \frac{(C_1 \times T_1) + (C_2 \times T_2) + (C_3 \times T_3) + (C_4 \times T_4) + (C_5 \times T_5)}{T_1 + T_2 + T_3 + T_4 + T_5}$$

$$\frac{400 + 1{,}200 + 20 + 100 + 600}{1 + 2 + 2 + 1 + 2} = \frac{2{,}320}{8} = 290 \text{ ppm}$$

36) We selected answer A because:

$$\frac{C_1}{T_1} + \frac{C_2}{T_2} + \frac{C_3}{T_3} = \text{exposure}$$

$$\frac{3}{4} + \frac{4}{8} + \frac{2}{\text{no limit}} = 1.25 \text{ is} > 1 \text{ exposure not allowed}$$

37) We selected answer B because:

Step 1: Determine the concentration of CO in the container.

$$\frac{2.5 \text{mL}}{190 \text{ L}} \times \frac{1 \text{ L}}{1{,}000 \text{ mL}} = 0.000013158$$

Step 2: Convert to ppm

$$0.000013158 \times 1{,}000{,}000 = 13.158 \text{ ppm}$$

38)   We selected answer C because:

Step 1:   Determine weight of accumulated material.

$$0.00\,4442\text{ g}$$
$$-0.00\,3422\text{ g}$$
$$\overline{0.00102\text{ g}}$$

Step 2:   Convert to desired units: mg.

$$\frac{0.00102\text{ g}}{1} \times \frac{1{,}000\text{ mg}}{1\,\text{g}} = 1.02\text{ mg}$$

Step 3:   Determine sample volume.

$$\frac{1.8\text{ L}}{1\text{ min}} \times \frac{4.33\text{ hr}}{1} \times \frac{60\text{ min}}{1\text{ hr}} = 468\text{ L}$$

Step 4:   Determine concentration in desired units.

$$\frac{1.02\text{ mg}}{468\,\text{L}} \times \frac{1000\text{ L}}{\text{m}^3} = 2.18\text{ mg/m}^3$$

39) We selected answer C because:

$$\frac{P_1\ V_1}{T_1} = \frac{P_2\ V_2}{T_2}$$

$$\frac{P_1}{T_1} = \frac{P_2}{T_2}$$

$$\frac{12.5}{515} = \frac{P_2}{580}$$

$$P_2 = \frac{12.5 \times 580}{515} = 14 \text{ psi}$$

40) We selected answer B because:

Double insulated equipment does not require a grounding conductor because of the extra protection provided by the additional insulation. Double insulation does not provide absolute protection (eg; a double insulated tool could still cause severe electrical shock if dropped in water).

41) We selected answer D because:

Training for powered industrial truck operators, good practice would indicate that refresher training is required periodically. However it is required that operators are evaluated at least every three years.

42) We selected answer C because:

Of the techniques listed for answers in this question, Job Safety Analysis would be the least effective. JSA tends to be too task oriented to be used successfully in a very complex operation. Fault Tree Analysis is excellent for scaling down huge complex systems, although the tree itself becomes fairly complex. Multilinear Events Sequencing (MES) is an accident investigation tool developed by Ludwig Benner Jr. of the National Transportation Safety Board and used extensively in aircraft mishap investigation. MES is a flow-charting methodology that, as the name implies, puts pertinent events in sequence. The attribute that really makes MES a star performer is the addition of a time line thus allowing duration, interval and sequence dimensions to be visualized, a concept very useful in accident investigation. Failure Modes and Effects Analysis was originally a reliability tool developed to allow predictions for the reliability of complex systems. It uses a tabular format to identify failures and the effect on the overall system. It is an excellent tool for spotting single point failures, but does not include any human interface.

43) We selected answer B because:

The National Fire Protection Association publishes several standards on fire extinguishers, however, many local jurisdictions have adopted the Uniform Fire Code in lieu of the NFPA standards. OSHA also has requirements for selection and placement of fire protection equipment.

44) We selected answer D because:

There are a number of Health & Safety Laws on the books today; however, the following are of particular interest to Health & Safety Practitioners taking the OHST examination

- Clean Air Act
- Clean Water Act
- Comprehensive Environmental Response, Compensation, And Liability Act (Superfund)
- Federal Insecticide, Fungicide And Rodenticide Act (FIFRA)
- Hazardous Materials Transportation Act (HMTA)
- National Environmental Policy Act (NEPA)
- Occupational Safety And Health Act (OSHA)
- Resource Conservation And Recovery Act (RCRA)
- Safe Drinking Water Act
- Superfund Amendments And Reauthorization Act 1986 (SARA)
- Toxic Substances Control Act (TSCA)

You should become familiar with the basic provisions of these important laws. Detailed analysis is not required. However, you should be able to distinguish between basic tenets.

45)   We selected answer D because:

The Federal Coal Mine Health and Safety Act was enacted in 1969. The Occupational Health and Safety Act was enacted in 1970. The Toxic Substance Control Act was enacted in 1976. The Metal and Non-metallic Mine Safety Act was enacted in 1966.

46)   We selected answer C because:

A pH of less than 7.0 indicates that the contents are acidic. A pH of more than 7.0 would indicate an alkaline cargo. A pH of 7 is considered neutral.

47)   We selected answer D because:

The Resource Conservation and Recovery Act (RCRA) requires that all waste be classified prior to handling. The waste is considered hazardous if it meets certain conditions or exhibits certain characteristics including tests for:

- Ignitability
- Corrosivity
- Reactivity
- Toxicity

48)   We selected answer D because:

According to 40 CFR 264 Subpart B, answers A, B and C are required.

49)   We selected answer D because:

The only agent listed that is rated for Class A firefighting is selection "D" Ammonium Phosphate, which is rated as an A:B:C extinguisher. Purple

K is Potassium Bicarbonate and is well known as an effective agent for flammable liquid fires, it is often used in combination with AFFF. Halon 1301, a halogenated agent, and the dry chemical potassium chloride is rated only B:C. Of the multi-purpose dry chemicals, monoammonium-phosphate-base is by far the most common and although considered non-toxic will cause irritation if breathed for extended periods. Another problem with ammonium phosphate is corrosion. The agent is acidic and when mixed with even minuscule amounts of water will corrode most metals, so immediate cleanup is very important.

50) We selected answer D because:

Assuming that the atmosphere in the confined space is oxygen deficient (worst case) the only appropriate choice is the Self Contained Breathing source.

51) We selected answer A because:

We believe the best instrument would be the Combustible Gas Indicator with Oxygen sensor. This would allow the OHST to rapidly determine the presence or lack of oxygen. Obviously, one would not make an entry into an unknown area such as this without appropriate provisions for rescue and a self-contained breathing apparatus.

52) We selected answer D because:

A pH of more than 7.0 indicates that the contents are a base or alkaline. A pH of less than 7.0 would indicate an acidic cargo. A pH of 7 is considered neutral.

53) We selected answer C because:

1910.120(p)(8)(iii)(A)

Training for emergency response employees shall be completed before they are called upon to perform in real emergencies. Such training shall include the elements of the emergency response plan, standard operating procedures the employer has established for the job, the personal protective equipment to be worn and procedures for handling emergency incidents.

Exception #1: an employer need not train all employees to the degree specified if the employer divides the work force in a manner such that a sufficient number of employees who have responsibility to control emergencies have the training specified, and all other employees, who may first respond to an emergency incident, have sufficient awareness training to recognize that an emergency response situation exists and that they are instructed in that case to summon the fully trained employees and not attempt control activities for which they are not trained.

54) We selected answer A because:

The GHS symbols have been incorporated into pictograms for use on the GHS label. Pictograms include the harmonized hazard symbols plus other graphic elements, such as borders, background patterns or colors which are intended to convey specific information. For transport, pictograms will have the background, symbol and colors currently used in the UN Recommendations on the Transport of Dangerous Goods, Model Regulations. For other sectors, pictograms will have a black symbol on a white background with a red diamond frame. A black frame may be used for shipments within one country. Where a transport pictogram appears, the GHS pictogram for the same hazard should not appear.

GHS Pictograms and Hazard Classes		
▪ Oxidizers	▪ Flammables ▪ Self Reactives ▪ Pyrophorics ▪ Self-Heating ▪ Emits Flammable Gas ▪ Organic Peroxides	▪ Explosives ▪ Self Reactives ▪ Organic Peroxides

• Acute toxicity (severe)	• Corrosives	• Gases Under Pressure
• Carcinogen • Respiratory Sensitizer • Reproductive Toxicity • Target Organ Toxicity • Mutagenicity • Aspiration Toxicity	• Environmental Toxicity	• Irritant • Dermal Sensitizer • Acute toxicity (harmful) • Narcotic Effects • Respiratory Tract Irritation

55) We selected answer D because:

Anthropometry is defined as the collection of information concerning both static and dynamic body measurements. *Automation* is a common synonym for any technological change involving the work place. *Autokinesis* refers to a form of disorientation where a fixed light appears to move against a dark background. *Autotrophic* is related to the study of biology and deals with utilizing only inorganic materials as a food source. This of course has little to do with ergonomics.

56) We selected answer C because:

1 Atom of Carbon = 12, 1 Atom of Oxygen = 16, 2 Atoms of Chlorine = 70

Molecular Weight = 98
70 / 98 = 71%

57) We selected answer C because:

One torr is equal to a pressure of 1 mm of mercury. It is named after the inventor of the mercury barometer.

58) We selected answer A because:

Lead sulfide plus hydrochloric acid yields lead chloride and hydrogen sulfide.

59) We selected answer A because:

Distance = Speed × Time

HINT: MPH × 1.47 = Feet per second

D = (45 × 5280 / 60 × 60) × 0.75 = 49.5 ft
                    OR
D = 45 × 1.47 × 0.75 = 49.6 ft

Convert to meters -- 50 ft × 0.3048 = 15.24 meters

60) We selected answer D because:

The training objective must be firmly established before a training program is undertaken.

61) We selected answer D because:

Boyle's Law expresses a very interesting relationship between the pressure and volume of a gas. It is stated as follows: The volume of a gas varies inversely as the pressure, provided the temperature remains constant. This means that if a quantity of gas has its pressure doubled, the volume becomes half of what it originally was.

62) We selected answer C because:

$$\frac{3.7 \times 10^{10}\, d}{1\,\sec} \times \frac{60\,\sec}{1\,\min} = 2.22 \times 10^{12}$$

63) We selected answer B because:

$$X = 9 - Y$$

$$3(9 - Y) - 2Y = 7$$

$$27 - 3Y - 2Y = 7$$

$$-5Y = 7 - 27$$

$$-5Y = -20$$

$$Y = 4$$

64) We selected answer A because:

The International System of Units (SI) adopted in April 1964, uses the name Celsius to indicate the temperature designation formerly known as Centigrade.

65) We selected answer C because:

$$5X - 7 = 3X - 3$$

$$5X = 3X + 4$$

$$2X = 4$$

$$X = 2$$

66) We selected answer D because:

The formula to convert is: $t_K = t_c + 273.16$. This answer is given in the Formulae, Equations, Constants and Conversions handout distributed for your use at the OHST exam. The same information is included in the complete guide to the OHST available from the BCSP.

67) We selected answer A because:

The *Loss Control Engineering Manual* published by A.M. Best Company contains definitions of most industrial types as well as the types of common losses that each class experiences.

68) We selected answer C because:

A benzene ring has 6 carbon atoms.

69) We selected answer B because:

A canopy generally can be used only as a receiving hood over hot processes to collect the gases and vapors rising into the hood. However, a canopy cannot be used when workers must lean over the tank or process because workers will breathe the contaminated air as the contaminants rise.

70) We selected answer B because:

$1 \text{ m}^3 = $ **1000 Liters**

71) We selected answer D because:

Building codes are designed to protect the future occupants of the building and offer little protection for the actual construction workers. Because codes attempt to predict the future use of the building they are considered the *absolute minimum protection* requirements.

72) We selected answer B because:

Respirable air under suitable pressure should be delivered to each respirator at a volume of at least 6 CFM.

73) We selected answer B because:

ANSI/ASME A17.1 concerns "Elevators, Escalators, and Moving Walks. "ANSI Z89.1 "Protective Headwear for Industrial Workers. "ANSI Z87.1 "Practice for Occupational and Educational Eye and Face Protection. "ANSI Z16.1 "Method of Recording and Measuring Work Injury Experience."

74) We selected answer D because:

Training of employees may not be required by every citation issued by OSHA.

75) We selected answer D because:

ANSI Z87.1 deals with Occupational and Educational Eye and Face Protection. *ANSI Z16.1* concern Uniform Recordkeeping for Occupational Injuries and Illnesses. *ANSI/ASME A12.1* is the standard for Floor and Wall Openings, Railings, and Toeboards. **ANSI Z89.1** is the authority on Protective Headgear for Industrial Workers.

76) We selected answer C because:

The CFRs are organized under 50 titles each dealing with broad subject areas of federal regulation. Relevance to the OHST examinations are:

CFR	Subject
10	Energy
14	Aeronautics and space
16	Consumer protection
23	Highways
29	Labor
40	Protection of the environment
42	Public health
49	Transportation

77)   We selected answer A because:

Washing with solvent is not a recommended practice and has a high probability of creating dermatoses.

78)   We selected answer A because:

CONTAMINANT	COLOR
Ammonia Gas	Green
Organic Vapors	Black
Carbon Monoxide Gas	Blue
Acid Gas and Organic Vapors	Yellow

79)   We selected answer B because:

Of the various methods available to the Occupational Health and Safety Technologist, *Engineering* controls are by far the preferred method. This would include initial design or by using the techniques of substitution, ventilation or isolation. *Administrative* controls that provide control of the worker's exposure are next in prevention value. *Personal Protective*

Equipment is the last resort to provide worker protection.

80)   We selected answer B because:

ANSI Z88.2 "Respirator Protection Factors" is to be used for guidance in the selection of respirators when complying with OSHA 1910.134 "Respiratory Protection". ANSI Z88.2 establishes some Protection Factors based on Qualitative or Quantitative fit testing. The chart below shows some information on various types of respirators.

TYPE OF RESPIRATOR	Respirator Protection Factors		
	Qualitative	Quantitative	IDLH
Particulate-filter, Vapor or gas, quarter or half mask. Includes combination filters.	10	Per-individual max of 100	NO
Particulate-filter, Vapor or gas, full face piece. Includes combination filters.	100	Per-individual max of 100	NO
Powered particulate-filter, Vapor or gas, full face piece any respiratory inlet covering.	No test required due to positive pressure. Max protection is 3000 with high efficiency filter.		NO
Air-line, demand, quarter or half mask face piece with or without escape provisions.	10	Per-individual must be less than IDLH	NO
Air-line, demand, full face piece with or without escape provisions.	100	Per-individual must be less than IDLH	NO
Air-line, continuous-flow or pressure-demand type any face piece. Includes helmet, hood, or suit, without escape provisions.	No test required due to positive pressure. Cannot exceed IDLH concentration.		NO
Air-line, continuous-flow or pressure-demand type any face piece. Includes helmet, hood, or suit, with escape provisions.	No test required due to positive pressure. Max protection factor is 10,000.		YES
SCBA, demand type, open circuit or negative pressure type closed circuit, full face piece.	100	Per-individual must be less than IDLH	NO
SCBA, pressure demand type, open circuit or positive pressure closed circuit, any facepiece.	No test required due to positive pressure. Max PF is 10,000.		YES

81)   We selected answer C because:

Grab samples are taken to measure the airborne concentration of a substance over a short time period (usually less than 5 min). Personal or area grab samples are used to identify peak or ceiling concentrations.

Grab samples alone are rarely used to estimate an employee's eight-hour time-weighted average exposure. This is because they do not account for the time between samples. However, they can be used as a screening method to determine whether more extensive sampling is needed.

82) We selected answer D because:

Ventilation does *not* control radiant heat.

83) We selected answer B because:

The purpose of local exhaust ventilation is to remove the air contaminants at the source not to dilute them.

84) We selected answer C because:

Dilution ventilation lowers the concentration of a contaminant by adding air to the general work area. Since the air is added to the general work area it will not effectively control exposure to a toxic or highly toxic substance used in a specific location.

85) We selected answer D because:

The following comparison is offered:

FOR THE SAME PROTECTION

Lead thickness required	0.3 inch
Sheet steel thickness required	1.3 inches
Concrete thickness required	2.7 inches
Water thickness required	8.3 inches

86) We selected answer C because:

Safety cans are required to be constructed of fire resistive materials, contain a flame arrestor and a self-closing cover, and be sized to prevent tipping. A fusible link that melts at a pre-determined temperature is not required.

87) We selected answer C because:

During respirator fit testing test subjects are asked to read the *Rainbow Passage*. This particular passage is selected, because it will result in a wide range of facial movements, and thus provide a good check of the respirator fit.

88) We selected answer D because:

Dilution ventilation is generally restricted to the following conditions:

- Small quantities of contaminant are released into the workplace air and at fairly uniform rates.
- The workplace contaminants are of low toxicity.
- Dilution ventilation will not cause corrosion or damage to equipment in the work area.
- There is enough room to allow air movement to dilute the contaminant to a low level.
- Dilution air can be discharged to the atmosphere without causing community environmental concerns.

89) We selected answer B because:

The term used to indicate the volume of air inhaled and exhaled in a normal human breath (500 cm^3) is *tidal volume*. The total amount of air that can be inhaled and exhaled during forced respiration is the *vital volume*. *Supplemental air* is the difference between tidal air and the maximum that can be exhaled. *Residual volume* is that amount of air that remains in our lungs no matter how hard we exhale (about 1500 cm^3).

90) We selected answer D because:

Fabric collectors are noted for the efficient removal of particles up to

99% with 0.5 μm particles. All of the other selections are true - fabric collectors can certainly be a fire or explosive hazard due to the concentrations present, they can be hard to clean and in many applications the major disadvantage is that they do not work well with moist gas.

91)   We selected answer D because:

Several precautions are generally employed in ovens that may contain dangerous concentrations of flammable gases. These precautions are necessary to prevent ignition of vapors during start up. The most common precaution is a timed pre-ignition purge that will ensure that 25% of the Lower Flammable Limit will not be exceeded. This pre-ignition purge is required after each shutdown of the recirculating or exhaust fans. Normally at least 4 cubic feet of fresh air per cubic foot of oven volume will be introduced during the purge cycle.

92)   We selected answer B because:

The use of a gas mask is permissible in an IDLH atmosphere due to the presence of a toxic contaminant for escape only.

93)   We selected answer B because:

This question seeks a situation that would *most likely* cause immediate functioning of a magnetic circuit breaker. The situation that qualifies is a line-to-line short. Undersize wiring would most likely result in an overload sufficient to operate the circuit breaker but only after a period of time (unless the wiring was grossly undersized). A 20% overload *might* operate the circuit breaker depending on other conditions. A ground fault would not operate the circuit breaker unless the ground fault resulted in a overload.

94)   We selected answer C because:

Protective creams sometimes called "Barrier" creams serve to inhibit contact with solvents in the work place. The use of protective creams is very controversial, however most of the current Safety and Health literature indicates that used properly these creams are useful. The cream must be used correctly to be effective which means it must be applied on clean skin at the beginning of the work shift, removed at lunch, reapplied after lunch, again in the afternoon, and removed at the close of the work shift.

95)   We selected answer D because:

Double insulation cannot prevent conductive paths in extremely wet locations.

96)   We selected answer A because:

Carpal tunnel syndrome involves an injury to the *median* nerve where the nerve is compressed due to inflammation in the carpal tunnel. The little finger is not served by the *median* nerve and therefore is not affected.

97)   We selected answer C because:

Damage to the eyes from ultraviolet radiation is much more violent than those of the visible or infrared, a severe burn can be produced with little or no warning and significant damage to the lens of the eye can occur.

98)   We selected answer B because:

According to the National Safety Council, the primary reason for safety training is to focus on behavior change.

99)   We selected answer A because:

The development and establishment of training objects must by necessity be one of the first steps taken in the development of any training program.

100) We selected answer B because:

The question accurately states the definition of toxicity.

Self-Assessment Exam Three Questions

1) A company decides to reflect the worker's compensation losses in terms of profits. The profit margin is 2.5% on each unit sold. What is the gross sales volume needed to offset $90,000 of worker's compensation costs?
   A) $600,000
   B) $3,000,000
   C) $3,600,000
   D) $30,000,000

2) Which of the following elements of a respirator maintenance program is **not** required?
   A) Inspection.
   B) Cleaning.
   C) Repair.
   D) Selection and Purchase.

3) Which of the following is **not** considered to be a significant external radiation hazard?
   A) Alpha.
   B) Beta.
   C) Gamma or X-Ray.
   D) Neutron.

4) A motor vehicle is traveling at 60 miles per hour, how many feet per second does this equal?
   A) 66 feet/second.
   B) 77 feet/second.
   C) 88 feet/second.
   D) 99 feet/second.

5)   Which of the following properties of activated carbon make it a good
     sample collecting or filtering medium?
     A)   Small surface area.
     B)   Is self cleaning over short period of time.
     C)   High adsorbency for gases, vapors.
     D)   High absorbency of the carrier gas only.

6)   What is the audible range for an average young person with unimpaired
     hearing?
     A)   Below 20 Hz.
     B)   Above 20,000 Hz.
     C)   Between 20 - 20,000 Hz.
     D)   Between 50 - 30,000 Hz.

7)   During total mass sampling, which of the following filters is used when
     gravimetric procedures are employed?
     A)   MCEF.
     B)   Glass fiber.
     C)   PVC.
     D)   Polycarbonate.

8)   Having an R number below 2000 implies what about flow characteristics
     in a ventilation system?
     A)   Laminar flow.
     B)   Turbulent flow.
     C)   Too fast for round ducts.
     D)   2000 is the breaking point for square ducts.

9)   Which of the following **best** describes the term "gravimetric"?
     A)   Absorbs water.
     B)   Reacts with water.
     C)   Measurement by weight.
     D)   Measurement by amount.

10) Which of the following **best** describes the current definition of breathing zone?
- A) A sphere 2 feet in diameter centered on the head.
- B) A sphere 2.2 feet in diameter centered on the head.
- C) A hemisphere 6-9 inches in radius and forward of the shoulders.
- D) A hemisphere 9-18 inches in radius and centered on the shoulder.

11) To be classified as a fiber, the aspect ratio (length to diameter) must be greater than:
- A) 1 to 1.
- B) 2 to 1.
- C) 3 to 1.
- D) 4 to 1.

12) Which of the following is the **best** definition of isokinetic conditions?
- A) Equal speeds in a ventilation system.
- B) Balance of gases in a stack.
- C) Primary calibration method for packed towers.
- D) Balance of probe air to stack air.

13) Which of the following would be the instrument of choice when measuring ventilation air flow involving corrosive gasses?
- A) Swinging vane anemometer.
- B) Heated thermocouple anemometer.
- C) Pitot tube.
- D) Rotating vane anemometer.

14) Which of the following is true concerning electrically operated handheld power tools?
- A) All power tools must be grounded.
- B) Double and triple insulated tools do not need to be grounded.
- C) Power operated tools must be connected to a GFCI when used outdoors.
- D) Grounding or GFCIs are required on construction sites.

15) In which case should an electrical branch circuit be protected by a
Ground Fault Circuit Interrupter (GFCI)?
   A) When used in an industrial environment.
   B) If extremely long extension cords are normally used.
   C) Adjacent to wet locations such as swimming pools.
   D) In all outside locations.

16) Assuming all other conditions would remain constant, which of the
following ventilation ducts would have the **most** resistance?
   A) 4 inch.
   B) 6 inch.
   C) 8 inch.
   D) 12 inch.

17) Which of the following is **not** a characteristic of a centrifugal fan?
   A) High volume with a low pressure drop.
   B) Low space requirement.
   C) Often used with particle laden air.
   D) Low to medium noise.

18) What is the predominant frequency to be expected from a fan, which is
direct driven at 4800 rpm, and delivers 2400 cfm at 0.25 in. water? The
fan has 60 backward curved blades.
   A) 3700 Hz.
   B) 3600 Hz.
   C) 2400 Hz.
   D) 4800 Hz.

19) The proper slant for a portable straight ladder is _____ feet vertical to
feet horizontal.
   A) 12 to 6 feet.
   B) 12 to 5 feet.
   C) 12 to 4 feet.
   D) 12 to 3 feet.

20) In ventilation hood design, the function of the slot in a slot hood is to:
   A) Increase capture velocity.
   B) Provide greater static pressure per horsepower.
   C) Obtain proper air distribution.
   D) Decrease capture velocity.

21) The explosimeter or combustible gas indicator operates on which of the following principles?
    A) Adsorption.
    B) Absorption.
    C) Latent heat of vaporization.
    D) Heat of combustion.

22) Which of the following statements is **not** true about the static pressure in a ventilation system?
    A) Static Pressure is measured parallel to the direction of flow.
    B) Static Pressure tends to collapse the duct in an exhaust system.
    C) Static Pressure acts in all directions.
    D) Static Pressure is a part of Total Pressure.

23) Which of the following does **not** require an equipment grounding conductor?
    A) A double reverse delta electrical system.
    B) A double insulated hand tool.
    C) A circuit that is protected with circuit breakers.
    D) A system with a wye connected transformer.

24) In the practice of Safety and Health, training is often offered as a universal solution. However, safety and health training should be targeted to real problems. Training should only be recommended as the solution to problems where increased knowledge or skill is needed or where required by directive. Which of the following **best** describes the reason or objective for after training testing?
    A) To weed out weak performers.
    B) To spot workers who have "attitude" problems.
    C) To spot weakness in the training program.
    D) To allow the students to see how much they learned.

25) For a potential laser exposure with an intensity of 1 watt/cm^3, what is the recommended optical density for laser glasses?
    A) 5.
    B) 6.
    C) 7.
    D) 8.

26) When the vapor pressure of a liquid is greater than the atmospheric pressure, this is known as the:
   A) Flash point (closed cup).
   B) Flash point (open cup).
   C) Boiling point.
   D) Freezing point.

27) Respiratory protection equipment is tested and approved by which of the following agencies?
   A) MSHA.
   B) OSHA.
   C) DOT.
   D) NIOSH.

28) Workers of which industry are affected by the disease silicosis?
   A) Government workers.
   B) Iron workers.
   C) Coal miners.
   D) Quartz miners.

29) Which of the following sound frequency ranges is generally considered to be the **most harmful** to hearing, especially the speech range?
   A) 37.5- 500 Hz.
   B) 1000-4000 Hz.
   C) 8000-16000 Hz.
   D) 16000-32000 Hz.

30) The inverse square law as applied to illumination states: The light intensity varies _____ with the _____ of the distance between source and surface.
   A) Directly, square.
   B) Inversely, square.
   C) Directly, ratio.
   D) Indirectly, ratio.

31) Which of the following is a characteristic of heat stroke?
- A) Lowered body temperature.
- B) Elevated body temperature.
- C) Normal body temperature.
- D) Profuse sweating.

32) Which of the following is the largest source of error when using colorimetric sampling devices?
- A) Charcoal packed too tight.
- B) Channeling.
- C) Temperature extremes.
- D) Interference from other contaminants.

33) Which of the following is the **best** statement concerning interchanging colorimetric tubes obtained from various manufacturers?
- A) Interchanging tubes is never permitted.
- B) Interchanging tubes is always permitted.
- C) Interchanging tubes is sometimes permitted.
- D) Interchanging tubes is allowed as long as the pump quantities are the same.

34) What are the three parts of a learning objective?
- A) Opening, body, close.
- B) Part 1, part 2, part 3.
- C) Pretest, lecture, posttest.
- D) Behavior, condition, degree.

35) When taking ventilation measurements and because the air flow in the cross-section of a duct is not uniform, it is necessary to obtain an average by measuring VP at points in a number of equal areas in the cross-section. The usual method is to measure along two paths that are at right angles to each other, this is called the?
- A) Pitot Traverse Method.
- B) Ventilation Measurement Method.
- C) Tuve Method.
- D) Burton Method.

36) A special case of tendosynovitis that occurs in the abductor and extensor tendons of the thumb where they share a common sheath. This condition often results from combined forceful gripping and hand twisting, as in wringing cloths and is called?
   A) Epicondylitis.
   B) Cubital Tunnel syndrome.
   C) Carpal Tunnel syndrome.
   D) DeQuervain's syndrome.

37) Which of the following would be the instrument of choice when checking an electrical equipment ground?
   A) Split-core ammeter.
   B) Polarity testing device.
   C) Impedance testing device.
   D) Volt-ohm meter.

38) A storage tank contains 18 cm of pooled hexane, which has a vapor pressure of 150 mm Hg. What is the maximum possible concentration of hexane vapor within the tank?
   A) 250 ppm.
   B) 20,000 ppm.
   C) 35,000 ppm.
   D) 197,368 ppm.

39) Harmful agents enter the human body in a variety of ways, which of the following is the **most common** route of entry?
   A) Skin Absorption.
   B) Ingestion.
   C) Inhalation.
   D) Puncture wounds.

40) Which of the following is **most correct** concerning a rigged object subject to the sudden movement of a hoisting apparatus during a hoisting operation?
   A) The load should be padded.
   B) The load will not be affected.
   C) Stresses will be increased in the rigging.
   D) Safety factors are based on the increased stresses caused by such operations.

41) Which of the following is the **best** description of Smoke?
    A)   Suspension of liquid particles formed by condensation.
    B)   Suspension of liquid or solid particles in air.
    C)   Aerosol formed from combustion of organic material.
    D)   Particulate material in air.

42) In industrial ventilation work a pitot traverse is often used to gain accurate measurements of the average duct velocity. However, a rule of thumb sometimes used, indicates that "the average duct velocity is about _____ percent of the centerline velocity".
    A)   60%
    B)   75%
    C)   80%
    D)   90%

43) Which of the following poses the **most common** exposure to ultraviolet radiation?
    A)   Stick welding.
    B)   Black Light.
    C)   Direct Sunlight.
    D)   Sun Guns.

44) Which of the following gases is **most likely** to be formed during welding operations conducted in close proximity to a tank of heated trichloroethylene?
    A)   Phosgene.
    B)   Carbon Monoxide.
    C)   Carbon Dioxide.
    D)   Oxides of Nitrogen.

45) The ratio of the mass of a unit volume of a substance to the mass of the same volume of a standard substance at a standard temperature is the definition of?
    A)   Unit Mass Comparison.
    B)   Specific Gravity.
    C)   Standard Deviation Measurement.
    D)   Laboratory Standard Measure.

46) While monitoring plant workers you discover that the TLV-STEL is being exceeded, for more than one hour, each work shift. Which of the following courses of action is appropriate?
   A) Continue monitoring and compute a new TWA.
   B) Recommend that the operation be curtailed immediately.
   C) Send the instrumentation for calibration.
   D) Continue as long as you do not exceed TLV-C values.

47) Which one of the following parts of the eye is **most likely** to suffer acute damage through exposure to infrared radiation?
   A) Fovea Centralis.
   B) Pupil.
   C) Retina.
   D) Sclera.

48) Lighting, radiation and sound are energy sources that follow the inverse square rule, which states: "The propagation of energy through space is inversely proportional to the square of the distance it must travel". Accordingly, if a lighting source has a illumination reading of 500 footcandles at 1 foot, what will the illumination be at 8 feet?
   A) 10 footcandles.
   B) 40 footcandles.
   C) 80 footcandles.
   D) 8 footcandles.

49) Film badge detectors are used to detect the presence of all of the following forms of ionizing radiation **except?**
   A) Gamma.
   B) Beta.
   C) X-Ray.
   D) Alpha.

50) What is the radius of a grinding wheel traveling at 3920 surface feet per minute and turning 1000 RPM?
   A) 12 inches.
   B) 15 inches.
   C) 6 inches.
   D) 7.5 inches.

51) Which of the following groups of hydrocarbons would have the greatest chance of **not** being flammable?
- A) Aliphatic Hydrocarbons.
- B) Aromatic Hydrocarbons.
- C) Halogenated Hydrocarbons.
- D) Ethers.

52) In welding practice, the term "GMAW" represents which of the following?
- A) Gas-Metal Atomizing Welding.
- B) Gas-Metal Arc Waste.
- C) Gas Metal Arc-Welding.
- D) Gas & Metallic Activated Welding.

53) According to OSHA, at what depth must a trench be shored or cut to the angle of repose?
- A) Greater than 4 feet.
- B) 5 feet or more.
- C) 4 feet.
- D) 6 feet or more.

54) According to OSHA, at what depth must a trench be provided with means of egress such as a stairway, ladder, ramp, etc.?
- A) Greater than 8 feet.
- B) 5 feet or more.
- C) 4 feet or more.
- D) 16 feet or more.

55) According to OSHA, what spacing is required between the required ladders in excavations classified as trenches?
- A) 50 feet.
- B) 100 feet.
- C) 25 feet.
- D) 30 feet.

56) A 1600 pound load is lifted with a 2 leg sling whose legs are at a 30 degree angle with the load. The stress on each leg of the sling is:
   A) 800 lbs.
   B) 1600 lbs.
   C) 2800 lbs.
   D) 3200 lbs.

57) If you measure 2000 cfm in a duct opening measuring 2 feet by 2 feet, what is the velocity of the air?
   A) 500 fpm.
   B) 8000 fpm.
   C) 200 fpm.
   D) 1600 fpm.

$$Q = A \times V$$

58) Doubling of any sound pressure corresponds to an increase of _____ dB in the sound pressure level?
   A) 0.6 dB.
   B) 6.0 dB.
   C) 3.0 dB.
   D) 0.3 dB.

59) If a chemical has an explosive range of 0.5 to 5%, what does this tell you about the LEL?
   A) 5,000 ppm is the LEL.
   B) 50,000 ppm is the LEL.
   C) 500 ppm is the LEL.
   D) None of the responses listed.

60) The elements Global Harmonized System (GHS) requires all of the following classification criteria **except?**
   A) Physical Hazards.
   B) Health and Environmental Hazards.
   C) Protective equipment requirements.
   D) Mixtures.

61) Compute the TWA concentration from the following measurement data: 0700-1000 hours @ 100 ppm---1000-1200 hours @ 200 ppm---1300-1400 hours @ 0 ppm and 1400-1600 hours @ 100 ppm.
   A) 100 ppm.
   B) 133.3 ppm.
   C) 112.5 ppm.
   D) 122 ppm.

62) Based on the allowable limits in the table below, if the noise in a work area was 95 dBA for 3 hours, 90 dBA for 4 hours and 85 dBA for 2 hours, what is the noise dose?
   A) 1.10
   B) .95
   C) 1.25
   D) 1.0

PERMISSIBLE NOISE EXPOSURES					
Hrs	dBA	Hrs	dBA	Hrs	dBA
8	90	3	97	1	105
6	92	2	100	0.5	110
4	95	1.5	102	0.25	115

63) Two machines are placed side-by-side, each machine produces 85 dB, what is the combined sound pressure level in decibels?
   A) 85 dB
   B) 170 dB
   C) 88 dB
   D) 127.5 dB

$$L_I = 10 Log \frac{I}{I_o} dB$$

64) The OSHA Permissible Exposure Limit (PEL) for asbestos fibers is an 8-hour TWA airborne concentration of 0.2 fiber per cubic centimeter of air as determined by the membrane filter method. What is the length-to-diameter ratio of the fibers to be counted using this method?
   A) 4 to 1.
   B) 3 to 1.
   C) 6 to 1.
   D) 5 to 1.

65) Calculate the sound pressure level in decibels given the following information. Actual sound pressure = 0.8n/m^2, Reference sound pressure = 0.00002 n/m^2.

  A) 82 dB.
  B) 88 dB.
  C) 92 dB.
  D) 102 dB.

$$L_p = 20 \log \frac{p}{p_o} \text{ dB}$$

66) ANSI Z16.2 is designed to provide a standardized method of recording certain accident facts. Which of the following would **not** be included under the provisions of ANSI Z16.2?

  A) Injury classifications.
  B) Hazardous Condition Classification.
  C) Workers' Compensation Rating.
  D) Unsafe Acts.

67) During sampling for Zinc fumes, a pump was calibrated at a flow rate of 2 L/min while connected to a representative sampler. A sample was taken in the field for 8 hours. The filter starting weight was 0.05551 g and the after sampling weight was 0.06661 g. The lab confirms the 70% of the material collected was ZnO. What is the concentration of ZnO in mg/m^3?

  A) 0.96 mg/m^3.
  B) 9.6 mg/m^3.
  C) 8.1 mg/m^3.
  D) 4.44 mg/m^3.

68) What is the volume of 7 liters of air at 30 inches Hg, when the pressure is changed to 25 inches Hg? Assume a constant temperature.

  A) 7.0 liters.
  B) 4.6 liters.
  C) 5.8 liters.
  D) 8.4 liters.

$$\frac{P_1 V_1}{T_1} = \frac{P_2 V_2}{T_2}$$

69) According to the OSHA Hazard Communication Standard, which of the following would **not** require employers to provide employees training on the hazardous chemicals in the workplace?

  A) Initial assignment.
  B) Resupply of chemicals.
  C) Change in job assignment with new chemicals.
  D) New chemical hazard in the work environment.

70) The OSHA requires employers to educate employees on Appendixes A & B of 29 CFR 1910.1025 when?
   A) Exposure can exceed the PEL.
   B) There is a potential of airborne lead at any level.
   C) The level exceeds the TLV-TWA.
   D) A citation is issued.

71) Which of the following is the **best** indicator of training effectiveness?
   A) Favorable Student Critiques.
   B) Correct Student Response to Questions.
   C) Increase in effectiveness of Job Performance.
   D) Testing meets expected norms.

72) Senior Management Officials can **best** support the Health and Safety training effort by?
   A) Hiring professional educators.
   B) Signing policy letters about H&S training importance.
   C) Showing active and sincere interest in the program.
   D) Talking about S&H at staff meetings.

73) During Health and Safety communications with workers, the main objective is to?
   A) Teach workers to understand what is being said.
   B) Provide a vehicle for suggestions.
   C) Teach workers to write and read well.
   D) Provide a safety message that will be understood and accepted by the workers.

74) Which of the following electrical devices would **most likely** to contain polychlorinated biphenyl (PCBs)?
   A) Transformers, capacitors, fluorescent light ballasts.
   B) Fuses, wiring and meters.
   C) Circuit breakers, panel board and unistrut.
   D) Meters, relays and switches.

75) An OSHA recordable includes which of the following?
  A) Medical treatment.
  B) Physician follow-up visit.
  C) First aid treatment.
  D) Over the counter medication.

76) OSHA requires serious accidents to be reported to the nearest area office of OSHA within 8 hours. The report must specifically include all of the following **except?**
  A) Number of fatalities or hospitalized employees.
  B) Contact person and phone number.
  C) Description of the incident.
  D) Most probable cause of the incident.

77) An employee at your plant strained her wrist. The plant RN had the employee use an elastic wristlet until the wrist had healed. How would this be recorded on the OSHA 300 Log?
  A) All other illnesses.
  B) Skin Disorder.
  C) Injury.
  D) Not recordable.

78) One training technique especially useful when dealing with craft employees during safety and health training is the case study. Which of the following is the **most correct** concerning a case study?
  A) Case studies must always involve fictitious situations or accidents so that no one group, or person will have hurt feelings.
  B) Case studies should be written and passed out as handouts to be most effective.
  C) Case studies are good problem-solving tools.
  D) Case studies involving real situations should only be used if they can be presented by the actual participants/victims.

79) When you develop the tests and evaluations for your training program, you should use all of the following guidelines **except?**
  A) Test items must be reliable.
  B) Evaluations are norm-referenced.
  C) Each test item must have criterion-related validity.
  D) The evaluation tool should be developed before the training

begins.

80) Which of the following training methods allows for the least amount of student-instructor interaction?
   A) Lecture.
   B) Role playing.
   C) Case study.
   D) Facilitated discussion.

81) You have been called on to determine the correct fire suppression agent for a fire involving a combustible metal used in your plant. Which agent would you choose?
   A) Green triangle with an A in the center.
   B) Red square with a B in the center.
   C) Blue circle with a C in the center.
   D) Yellow star with a D in the center.

82) The Life Safety Code includes the term exit in an overall definition of means of egress. A means of egress includes three parts, which are: the exit, the access, and the:
   A) Width of isles.
   B) Number of doors.
   C) Height of tread riser.
   D) Exit discharge with unobstructed path to the street.

83) Once you obtained your OHST, you must maintain your currency in the safety and health arena. This is monitored by the BCSP by the Continuance of Certification program. All the following are ways to obtain certification points **except?**
   A) Engaged in acceptable, professional safety practice for at least 25% of a 40 hour work week.
   B) Serving as an officer on approved technical/professional committees or safety organizations.
   C) Contributions to the safety body of knowledge through publications, presentations and patents.
   D) Drafting OHST examination questions at workshops or by submitting them individually.

84) If OHSTs were petitioning to the state to have only certified individual recognized as safety and health professionals, this would be an example of:
   A) Title Protection.
   B) Professional Registration.
   C) A Title Act.
   D) Professional Competence Standard.

85) The OHST certification is sponsored through the Board of Certified Safety Professionals (BCSP). The BCSP is sponsored by?
   A) ABIH & NSC.
   B) ABIH & AHMP.
   C) ASSE & ABIH.
   D) NSC & ASSE.

86) People in leadership positions influence ethical behavior primarily by?
   A) Professional ethics.
   B) Daily actions.
   C) Private affairs.
   D) Social acceptance.

87) A standard that is specific, that is, has application for a specific industry only is:
   A) A performance standard.
   B) A specification standard.
   C) A vertical standard.
   D) A horizontal standard.

88) What is the failure rate of a device that has four components connected in series? Each component has a failure rate of 0.05.
   A) 0.625
   B) 0.05×10^4
   C) 0.02
   D) 0.2

89) An elevated water tank produces a ground level pressure of 95 psi. How high is the tank?
   A)   About 255 feet.
   B)   About 65 feet.
   C)   About 40 feet.
   D)   About 220 feet.

90) Section 1910.1000 (Air Contaminants) of the General Industry Standard would be classified as what kind of standard?
   A)   Vertical.
   B)   Performance.
   C)   Specification.
   D)   Optional.

91) Accidents usually result from:
   A)   Personality factors.
   B)   Environmental factors.
   C)   Physical limitations.
   D)   Combinations of factors.

92) The **best** way to deal with minor infractions of work or safety rules?
   A)   Oral reprimand.
   B)   Written reprimand.
   C)   Ignore it.
   D)   Suspension.

93) All of the following compressed cylinders require safety relief devices **except?**
   A)   Oxygen.
   B)   Nitrogen.
   C)   Poison-A.
   D)   Argon.

94) Acclimatization to heat is generally achieved by requiring the employee to?
   A)   Work at 50% of the desired work rate.
   B)   Work at 75% of the desired work rate.
   C)   Work for two hours per day for one week.
   D)   Work for six hours per day for two months.

95) The use of testing during safety training provides an opportunity to determine the effectiveness of the education effort. Before and after testing is often used as a measure of effectiveness. Which of the following techniques is true concerning the "before and after testing" method?
    A) Before and after tests should be identical.
    B) Before and after tests should not be used.
    C) Before and after tests should cover the same areas but the questions should be phrased differently.
    D) Before and after tests should be very comprehensive to ensure that all areas requiring attention were covered.

96) All of the following are valid reasons for accident (mishap) investigation **except?**
    A) Prevent reoccurrence of similar events.
    B) Establish casual factors.
    C) Provide vehicle for discipline.
    D) Provide data for trend analysis.

97) Which of the following is generally **not** considered to be an indirect cost of accidents?
    A) Wages paid to fellow workers for loss of productivity.
    B) Cost of accident investigation team.
    C) Cost to train new worker.
    D) Cost of physical therapy.

98) Which of the following statements is in agreement with the domino theory of accident causation?
    A) All accidents have multiple causes.
    B) Improper training causes most accidents.
    C) An accident is symptomatic of a management error.
    D) An unsafe act or condition initiates the accident sequence.

99) The **primary** purpose for using On-the-Job training is:
    A) It is cost effective.
    B) More than one person can be trained at a time.
    C) Requires the minimum amount of time for total training.
    D) Allows the worker to produce during the training period.

100) You are the Safety Director of a textile plant that has received an OSHA inspection. You were cited for several violations and your citations have been received at the main plant. Which of the following actions is **most correct?**

  A) You must pay the fine within 15 working days.
  B) The workers must be allowed to see the citation.
  C) You must fix the discrepancy within 30 days.
  D) You must post the citations for at least three days.

Self-Assessment Exam Three Answers

1)   We selected answer C because:

$3,600,000 in gross sales at 2.5% profit margin is required to offset $90,000 in worker's compensation losses.

90,000 / 0.25 = 3,600,000

2)   We selected answer D because:

The respirator maintenance program should include inspection for defects, cleaning, disinfecting, provisions for storage, and repair. Selection and Purchase by definition do not belong to the "maintenance" program.

3)   We selected answer A because:

Alpha radiation is non-penetrating and is not considered an external hazard because of the protection provided by the outer layer of skin.

4)   We selected answer C because:

$$\frac{60 \times 5280}{60 \times 60} = 88 \text{ ft per sec}$$

HINT: 5280÷3600 = 1.47 (a constant that is often used in these types of problems)

$$60 \times 1.47 = 88 \text{ ft per sec}$$

5)   We selected answer C because:

Activated carbon is extremely porous and has a non-polar surface. It adsorbs molecules to its surface readily. When bathed in a non-polar solvent such as carbon disulfide the adsorbed molecules are easily removed and dissolved into the solvent.

6)   We selected answer C because:

Below 20 Hz is sub-audible, above 20,000 is ultrasonic. The average measured hearing range of an unimpaired person is 20-20,000 Hz.

7)   We selected answer C because:

Polyvinyl chloride (PVC) is widely used for gravimetric determination during mass sampling, i.e.; total dust, coal dust, respirable dust, etc. The other filters are not efficient because of the ability to retain water that affects the weighing process.

8)   We selected answer A because:

The Reynolds number is a dimensionless ratio used to predict if flow is turbulent or laminar. If the Reynolds number is less than 2000 the flow is laminar; if greater than 2100 the flow is turbulent.

9)   We selected answer C because:

The classic definition of gravimetric is the practice of measurement by weight. The OHST examination, and the safety and health profession, have historically used the term when referring to mass sampling techniques.

10)   We selected answer C because:

The preferred definition of Breathing Zone is a hemisphere forward of the shoulders with a radius of approximately 6 to 9 inches.

11) We selected answer C because:

Fibers are particles, which have a length that is at least three times its width.

12) We selected answer D because:

None of these answers are very descriptive. Iso means equal, kinetic means motion, and therefore isokinetic means equal motion. Isokinetic conditions when applied to OHST tasks typically means that the velocity of gas entering a sampling probe is equal to the sample stream. If the velocity of the sample stream is greater than the velocity entering the probe the contaminant will be oversampled. So obviously, if the velocity of the sample stream is less than the velocity entering the probe the contaminant will be undersampled.

13) We selected answer C because:

The pitot tube would be our instrument of choice. The pitot tube has several qualities that make it ideal for use under severe conditions. It has no moving parts, is extremely rugged, and withstands high temperature and corrosive atmospheres (when made of stainless steel).

14) We selected answer B because:

Double or Triple insulated tools do not require equipment grounding due to the extra protection provided by the insulation.

15) We selected answer C because:

There are many locations where GFCI are required. However, they are not required in all industrial application. Additionally, they generally do not function properly when protecting a circuit that is extremely long (250 feet as a rule) because of the capacitive leakage to ground in these circuits.

The use of a GFCI is very desirable when using electrical equipment outdoors especially if it is wet, but they are required by Article 680 of the National Electrical Code in and around swimming pools. A few locations where GFCI protection is required include:

- On outdoor receptacles in dwellings where there is grade level access.
- On bathroom receptacles in dwellings.
- On receptacles in dwelling garages (unless circuit includes clothes washers, freezers, garage-door openers etc.
- In kitchens within 6 feet of sinks or grounded metal case appliances.
- On construction sites.
- In and around swimming pools, spas etc.

Remember, the GFCI will not prevent a shock, it will render them relatively harmless if installed properly. It will not protect from direct line-to-line contact.

16) We selected answer A because:

Assuming the same velocity of air the smaller diameter ducts have higher friction losses and provide the most resistance to air flow. For example, a 4 inch duct, 14 foot long has the same resistance to flow as 40 foot of 10 inch duct.

17) We selected answer A because:

High volume and low pressure drop are characteristics of axial flow fans which are most commonly used for general ventilation or dilution ventilation work. Centrifugal fans are used against low to moderate static pressures such as encountered in heating and air conditioning work. These fans have low space requirements and are quiet. The paddle wheel or long shaving wheel is used with a medium tip speed for buffing exhaust, woodworking exhaust or when a heavy dust must pass through the fan.

18) We selected answer D because:

The predominant frequency is calculated by determining the number of times per second the blades pass a fixed point. So 4800 rpm = 80 revolutions per second. 80 rps x 60 blades = 4800 Hz.

19) We selected answer D because:

The safe procedure for setting up a ladder requires the base to be one-fourth the ladder length. 3/12 = 1/4

20) We selected answer C because:

Slot hoods are commonly used to provide uniform exhaust airflow, such as over the surface of a tank. **Points to remember:**
- The function of the slot is solely to obtain proper air distribution.
- Slot velocity does not contribute to capture velocity.
- The calculation of capture velocity involves exhaust volume and slot length, not slot velocity.

21) We selected answer D because:

If explosive meter or combustible gas indicator is of the hot wire type it causes an oxidation to take place, determines the deviation, and indicates a measurement based on the heat released.

22) We selected answer A because:

The static pressure is always measured perpendicular to the direction of flow.

23) We selected answer B because:

Double insulated equipment does not require a grounding conductor because of the extra protection provided by the additional insulation.

24)   We selected answer C because:

There are two objectives to after training testing. First, to see if the student has gained skill or knowledge in the subject area. Second, to assist the developer and instructor in evaluating the effectiveness of instruction. For example, if a significant percentage of the students in an average class cannot perform up to the specifications outlined in the lesson plans, then the instruction is simply not working. The problem could be the atmosphere, the instructional method, instruction techniques, the instructor, training material, etc. In any event, changes are in order. Effective training is a complex task, in which evaluation of the instruction is often overlooked.

25)   We selected answer C because:

Intensity, CW maximum Power Density (watts/cm^3)	Optical Density (OD)	Attenuation Factor
10^2	5	10^5
10^4	6	10^6
1	7	10^7
10	8	10^8

Source: 29 CFR 1926.102

26)   We selected answer C because:

When the vapor pressure of a liquid is greater than the atmospheric pressure, the material has reached its boiling point.

27)   We selected answer D because:

Within the United States, both NIOSH and MSHA test and approve respiratory protection.

28) We selected answer D because:

Quartz miners would be exposed to the fine quartz dust that can cause silicosis.

29) We selected answer B because:

The ear is most susceptible to noise in the range of 1000-4000 Hz.

30) We selected answer B because:

The inverse square law states that: The light intensity on a surface varies inversely with the square of the distance between the source and the surface.

31) We selected answer B because:

The symptoms of heat stroke include an elevated temperature and dry skin (not sweat).

32) We selected answer D because:

Interference from other substances in the sample air should always be a primary consideration, because the greatest single source of error in colorimetric sampling is interferences by other contaminants.

33) We selected answer A because:

The practice of interchanging colorimetric tubes is not permitted because it may lead to erroneous results. The primary considerations are the volume of the pump and the rate of the chemical reagents in the indicator tubes.

34) We selected answer D because:

According to the NSC there are four parts (ABCD), audience, behavior, condition and degree. However, some other experts only list the last three.

35) We selected answer A because:

According to the ACGIH *Industrial Ventilation* Manual, this is the definition of a Pitot Traverse.

36) We selected answer D because:

This is the definition of DeQuervain's syndrome.

37) We selected answer C because:

We prefer an impedance testing device that provides a measurement of total impedance (opposition to AC current) by injecting a high current spike onto the circuit under test. This device will identify those points of low thermal capacity that will cause high system resistance under load. The other instruments use a very small current and will not detect inadequate thermal capacity, which under high fault currents will cause overheating and possibly result in arcing fires.

38) We selected answer D because:

This is a partial pressure question. Using Dalton's Law - in a mixture of gases, each gas exerts pressure independently of the other gases present. The partial pressure of each gas is proportional to the amount of that gas in the mixture (percent by volume). So:

$$\frac{150}{760} \times 1,000,000 = 197,368 \text{ ppm}$$

*Note:The alternate solution using the "VP × 1300" rule of thumb yields:

$$150 \times 1300 = 195,000 \text{ ppm}$$

39) We selected answer C because:

Inhalation is the major route for industrial contaminants. Inhalation is significant not only because it is the most common path but because of the rapidity with which a toxic material can be absorbed in the lungs, or nasal passages, passed to the bloodstream, and reach the brain.

40) We selected answer C because:

The inertia of an object in motion that takes place when an increase or decrease in speed causes great increases in stress on the rigging. As a load line starts to move sudden accelerations can cause as much as twice the stress on the rigging as the actual load. This is why most rigging or hoisting instructions contain warnings or cautions about applying lifting forces in a slow and smooth manner.

41) We selected answer C because:

Historically, there have been questions on the examination concerning the definition of the following:

- Smoke - aerosol formed from combustion of organic material (0.01 - 0.5μm)
- Dust - Particulate material generated by a mechanical process (0.5 - 50 μm)
- Aerosol - Suspension of liquid or solid particles in air
- Mist - Suspension of liquid particles in air formed by condensation from vapor or by some mechanical process (40 - 400μm)
- Fume - Solid particle aerosol formed by condensation from the vapor state (0.001 - 0.2μm)

42) We selected answer D because:

Using the rule that the average duct velocity is about 90% of the centerline velocity is not a recommended practice. A pitot traverse is much preferred. This involves measuring the velocity at a number of points across the duct area since velocity distribution is not uniform within the duct. Often in working ventilation systems turbulent or stratified airflow is present throughout the system this makes any approximation very inaccurate.

43)   We selected answer C because:

Sunlight is the major source of ultraviolet radiation among the sources listed.

44)   We selected answer A because:

Cleaning with chlorinated solvents within the general area of welding operations can cause major hazards due to the creation of *phosgene gas*. A study conducted by NIOSH examined several cases of respiratory distress and pulmonary function impairment associated with phosgene poisoning. One case involved seven workers who complained of mild to severe respiratory distress, cough, chest constriction, and breathlessness while they performed gas metal arc welding. The source of the discomfort was found to be phosgene gas produced by vapors from an inadequately ventilated degreasing tank that contained trichlorethylene. The tank was located downstream almost 150 feet away from the welding bay. Trichlorethylene vapors had decomposed as a result of heat and ultraviolet radiation from the arc and created enough phosgene to poison these workers.

45)   We selected answer B because:

Specific Gravity is the measure of the mass of a given substance in comparison to a standard substance. If the material is liquid, water is used as the standard. If the material is gas, air is used as the standard substance.

46)   We selected answer B because:

TLV-STEL (*Threshold Limit Value - Short-Term Exposure Limit)* is the concentration to which workers can be exposed continuously for a short period of time without suffering from:

- Irritation
- Chronic or irreversible tissue damage
- Narcosis of sufficient degree to increase the likelihood of accidental injury, impair self-rescue or materially reduce work efficiency

The STEL is defined as a 15-minute TWA exposure, which should not be exceeded at any time during a workday even if the 8-hour TWA is within the TLV-TWA. Exposures above the TLV-TWA up to the STEL should generally be no longer than 15 minutes for no more than four times per shift. With at least one hour between excursions.

47)   We selected answer C because:

Infrared (IR) radiation passes easily through the cornea and the energy is absorbed by the lens and retina.

48)   We selected answer D because:

$$I_2 = I_1 \times \frac{(d_1)^2}{(d_2)^2}$$

$$I_2 = I_1 \times \frac{(1)^2}{(8)^2}$$

$$I_2 = 500 \times \frac{1}{64}$$

$$I_2 = 7.8 \text{ footcandles}$$

49) We selected answer D because:

Alpha radiation is a non-penetrating form of radiation. Alpha cannot be detected by the film badge, which requires penetration of the surface covering the film before a measure can be made.

50) We selected answer D because:

Step 1: Determine Circumference

$$C = \frac{SFM}{RPM}$$

$$C = \frac{3920}{1000}$$

$$C = 3.92 \ ft$$

Step 2: Determine Radius

$$R = \frac{C}{2\pi}$$

$$R = \frac{3.92 \ ft}{6.28}$$

$$R = .624 \ ft$$

$$R = 7.488 \ inches$$

51) We selected answer C because:

Hydrocarbons are compounds that contain atoms of carbon and hydrogen only. They are broadly classified into two types, that is; aliphatic and aromatic. *Aliphatic hydrocarbons* are subdivided into saturated and unsaturated compounds and include the alkanes: methane, ethane, propane and butane. *Aromatic hydrocarbons* are derivative of the parent compound benzene. *Ethers* are members of a class of organic compound in which an oxygen atom has bridged between two hydrocarbon groups. Aliphatic ethers are highly volatile and extremely flammable. Hydrocarbons that have been partially halogenated will burn, but generally with much less ease than their nonhalogenated analogs. The fully *halogenated* derivatives such as carbon tetrachloride are non-combustible.

52) We selected answer C because:

GMAW stands for Gas Metal Arc-Welding, which is a process that joins metals by heating them with an arc between continuous filler metal electrode and the work, shielding is obtained from an external supplied gas or gas mixture. The process is often called MIG or CO_2 welding. Because of the inherent safety and health hazards involved in the welding process the OHST examination has historically contained several questions on the different processes and the hazards associated with each.

53) We selected answer B because:

Excavations that are less than 5 feet in depth do not require shoring or sloping, if examination of the ground is conducted by a competent person, who finds no indication of a potential cave-in. The "angle of repose" is the angle at which soil will no longer slide, in this instance it means to slope to a flat enough of an angle to prevent the soil from sliding back into the ditch. A quick review of OSHA 1926.651 and 652 is in order prior to taking the OHST examination.

54) We selected answer C because:

Means of egress from trench excavations such as a stairway, ladder, ramp or other safe means of egress are required in trench excavations that are 4 feet or more in depth and located so as to require no more than 25 feet of lateral travel for workers. OSHA 1926.651.

55) We selected answer A because:

Means of egress from trench excavations such as a stairway, ladder, ramp or other safe means of egress are required in trench excavations that are 4 feet or more in depth and located so as to require **no more than 25 feet of lateral travel** for workers. Ladders placed every 50 running feet of trench would provide a maximum of 25 feet of travel in each direction, assuming an initial ladder at the start of the trench run. OSHA 1926.651.

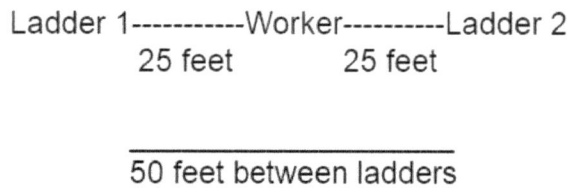

Ladder 1-----------Worker----------Ladder 2
     25 feet   25 feet

            _____
     50 feet between ladders

56) We selected answer B because:

$$\sin A = \frac{a}{c}$$

$$c = \frac{a}{\sin A}$$

$$c = \frac{800}{\sin 30}$$

$$c = 1600 \text{ lbs}$$

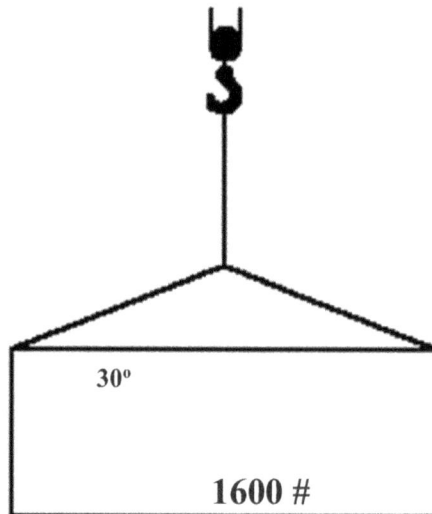

HINT: Double divided SLINGS are SIN full. Divide by two and then divide again by the SIN of the angle.

$$1600 / 2 / \sin 30 = 1{,}600 \text{ lbs}$$

57) We selected answer A because:

$$Q = A \times V$$

$$V = \frac{Q}{A}$$

$$V = \frac{2000 \text{ cfm}}{4 \text{ ft}^2}$$

$$V = 500 \text{ fpm}$$

58) We selected answer C because:

Doubling of any sound pressure level corresponds to an increase of 3 dB in the sound pressure level.

59) We selected answer A because:

The Lower Explosive Limit LEL is 0.5% or 5,000 ppm.

$0.5\% = .005$ then $.005 \times 1,000,000 = 5,000$ PPM

60) We selected answer C because:

The GHS hazard definitions are criteria-based and address three main classification criteria; Health and Environmental Hazards; Physical Hazards; and Mixtures. Classification is the starting point for hazard communication. It involves the identification of the hazard(s) of a chemical or mixture by assigning a category of hazard/danger using defined criteria. The GHS is designed to be consistent and transparent. It draws a clear distinction between classes and categories in order to allow for **"self classification"**. For many hazards a decision tree approach (e.g., eye irritation) is provided in the GHS Document. For several hazards the GHS criteria are semi-quantitative or qualitative. Expert judgment may be required to interpret these data. It is recommended that the person responsible for GHS implementation consult the GHS Document or "Purple Book" for more complete information.

61) We selected answer C because:

$$\text{TWA} = \frac{(C_1 \times T_1) + (C_2 \times T_2) + (C_3 \times T_3) + (C_4 \times T_4)}{T_1 + T_2 + T_3 + T_4}$$

$$TWA = \frac{300 + 400 + 0 + 200}{3 + 2 + 1 + 2} = \frac{900}{8} = 112.5 \text{ ppm}$$

62) We selected answer C because:

$$\frac{C_1}{T_1} + \frac{C_2}{T_2} + \frac{C_3}{T_3} = \text{dose}$$

$$\frac{3}{4} + \frac{4}{8} + \frac{2}{\text{no limit}} = 1.25$$

63) We selected answer C because:

When the sound pressure level expressed in decibels is doubled it will result in an increase of 3 dB.

$$L_I = 10 \text{Log} \frac{I}{I_o} \text{dB}$$

Step 1: Use the formula for sound level intensity.

The level increased 2 times the reference of 85 or 2 over 1.

$$L_I = 10 \times \text{Log} \frac{2}{1}$$

Log 2 times 10

$$L_I = 10 \times 0.3010$$

Results in a 3 dB increase

$$L_I = 3.01 \text{dB} \uparrow$$

Step 2: Add the increase to the reference number $85 + 3 = 88$ dB

64)   We selected answer B because:

To be considered asbestos fibers, the fibers counted must be longer than 5 micrometers and have a length-to-diameter ratio of at least 3 to 1.

65)   We selected answer C because:

$$L_p = 20 \log \frac{p}{p_o} \, dB$$

$$L_p = 20 \times \log \frac{0.8}{0.00002}$$

$$L_p = 20 \times 4.602$$

$$L_p = 92 \, dB$$

66)   We selected answer C because:

ANSI Z16.2 does not include any provisions for recording workers compensation information. The classifications that are included are:

- Nature of Injury
- Part of Body Affected
- Source of Injury
- Accident Type
- Hazardous Condition
- Agency of Accident
- Agency of Accident Part
- Unsafe Act

67)   We selected answer C because:

$$\begin{array}{r} 0.06661\,g \\ -\,0.05551\,g \\ \hline 0.0111\,g \end{array}$$

Step 1:   Determine weight of accumulated material and amount of ZnO

$$0.0111 \times 0.70 = 0.00777\,g$$

Step 2:   Convert to desired units

$$\frac{0.00777\,g}{1} \times \frac{1{,}000\,mg}{1\,g} = 7.77\,mg$$

Step 3:   Determine sample volume

$$\frac{2\,L}{1\,min} \times \frac{8\,hr}{1} \times \frac{60\,min}{1\,hr} = 960\,L$$

Step 4:   Determine concentration in desired units

$$\frac{7.77\,mg}{960\,L} \times \frac{1{,}000\,L}{m^3} = 8.1\,mg/m^3$$

68)   We selected answer D because:

$$\frac{P_1 V_1}{T_1} = \frac{P_2 V_2}{T_2}$$

$$P_1 V_1 = P_1 V_1$$

$$30 \times 7 = 25 \times V_2$$

$$V_2 = \frac{30 \times 7}{25}$$

$$V_2 = 8.4 \text{ liters}$$

69) We selected answer B because:

According to the OSHA Hazard Communication Standard (29 CFR 1910.1200), employers shall provide employees with information and training on hazardous chemicals in their work area:

- at time of initial assignment
- if transferred to a new assignment with new chemical hazards
- when a new chemical hazard is introduced into the work place

70) We selected answer B because:

The OSHA Lead Standard (29 CFR 1910.1025) requires that each employer who has a workplace in which there is a potential exposure to airborne lead at any level inform employees of the content of Appendixes to the standard. A training program with the participation of all employees is required for all employees who are subject to exposure to lead at or above the action level or where the possibility of skin or eye irritation exists.

71) We selected answer C because:

Job performance is the most effective and final measure of any training program.

72) We selected answer C because:

Management can best support any Health and Safety effort by showing active and sincere interest in the program. This support can take many forms, but it is vitally important that the message that reaches the company floor be consistent and sincere. If the boss really wants safety, so will the workers.

73) We selected answer D because:

The bottom line in any training or education effort is to provide a message that will be understood and acted on by the workers.

74)   We selected answer A because:

Polychlorinated biphenyl (PCBs) are found in certain electrical devices such as transformers, capacitors, fluorescent light ballasts, etc. as well as in heat transfer enclosures and investment casting waxes in foundries. In 1978, the EPA banned the use of PCBs in light ballasts, transformers and capacitors however it is still possible to find equipment containing PCBs.

75)   We selected answer A because:

Medical treatment must be logged as an OSHA recordable.

76)   We selected answer D because:

The requirement to establish a "most probable cause" on a 8 hour report is not realistic nor desirable as it encourages speculation. OSHA 1904.8, *Reporting of fatality or multiple hospitalization incidents* is quoted here for your information.

"(a) Within 8 hours after the death of any employee from a work-related incident or the in-patient hospitalization of three or more employees as a result of a work-related incident, the employer of any employees so affected shall orally report the fatality/multiple hospitalization by telephone or in person to the Area Office of the Occupational Safety and Health Administration (OSHA), U.S. Department of Labor, that is nearest to the site of the incident, or by using the OSHA toll-free central telephone number.

(b) This requirement applies to each such fatality or hospitalization of three or more employees that occurs within thirty (30) days of an incident.

(c) Exception: If the employer does not learn of a reportable incident at the time it occurs and the incident would otherwise be reportable under paragraphs (a) and (b) of this section, the employer shall make the report within 8 hours of the time the incident is reported to any agent or employee of the employer.

(d) Each report required by this section shall relate the following information: Establishment name, location of incident, time of the incident, number of fatalities or hospitalized employees, contact person, phone number, and a brief description of the incident."

77) We selected answer D because:

According to the 1904.7, "Using any non-rigid means of support, such as elastic bandages, wraps, non-rigid back belts, etc. (devices with rigid stays or other systems designed to immobilize parts of the body are considered medical treatment for recordkeeping purposes) is considered first-aid.

78) We selected answer C because:

The case study is an especially effective technique for safety and health training, since it often illustrates the multi-causal aspects of accidents as well as the tragic consequences. The case study is an excellent problem solving technique. Normally case studies are presented to a group that has the goal of evaluating the mistakes made in the situation and providing real world solutions. The technique is particularly effective when the group is allowed to come to the conclusion that they can benefit from the mistakes of other construction contractors and thus prevent accidents. Real mishaps are effective case studies and should be used as often as possible to add credibility to the technique, but one must be aware of the sensitivities involved in tragic accidents.

79) We selected answer B because:

Reliability is a measure of how well a test item discriminates the knowledge level of the participants.

Evaluations for training purposes are **NOT norm-referenced**. Norm-referencing means that how well a trainee scores depends on how well or how poorly other trainees perform.

Evaluations for training purposes **should always be criterion-referenced**. This means performance is measured against a pre-set standard. The test must measure what it is supposed to measure.

The evaluation tool should always be developed before training begins.

80) We selected answer A because:

The benefits of the lecture is that you can impart information to a large group in a relative short time, however this leaves little time or opportunity for interaction between the trainee and the instructor.

81) We selected answer D because:

The green triangle with an "A" is for ordinary combustible fires. "B" is for flammable liquids. "C" is electrical equipment. "D" is for fires involving certain combustible metals.

82) We selected answer D because:

A means of egress is a continuous path of travel from any point in a building or structure to the open air outside at ground level and consists of three separate and distinct parts; (1) the way of exit access; (2) the exit; and (3) the means of discharge from the exit.

83) We selected answer A because:

CM point rules are outlined in the Certification Maintenance Guide and include the following categories:

- Safety and Health Practice (35% of 30 hour week)
- Health & Safety Organization Membership
- Technical/Professional Committee Service, Safety & Health Organizations Offices
- Professional Publications, Papers, Technical Presentations and Patent
- Preparation of Examination Questions
- Professional Development Conferences
- Continuing Education Courses
- College or University Courses
- Academic Degrees
- Re-examination

84) We selected answer A because:

A Title Act is the method a state would choose to enact specific Title

Protection. The purpose of title protection according to an ASSE Position Statement is to "provide legal recognition to the profession of safety as well as provide assurance to the public that individuals representing themselves as being involved in the profession of safety **as safety professionals,** have met the listed minimum qualifications, thereby protecting the public health and safety from harm."

If an individual uses the OHST designation without first being certified by the BCSP, that individual may be barred from pursuing any BCSP certification and/or be sued.

85) We selected answer B because:

The BCSP is sponsored by the American Board of Industrial Hygiene and the Board of Certified Safety Professionals.

86) We selected answer B because:

Not only does management have to "talk the talk", they have to "walk the talk" if they expect the employees to believe that they really mean what they say.

87) We selected answer C because:

A vertical standard applies to a single industry. A specification standard demands precise compliance with exacting codes, frequently detailing exact specifications for materials, sizes, etc. A performance standard tells us that we must comply and leaves the details up to the industry.

88) We selected answer D because:

For components in series, the total failure rate is the sum of the individual components' failure rates

$$0.05 + 0.05 + 0.05 + 0.05 = 0.2$$

89) We selected answer D because:

$$psi = k \times H \quad H = Height \quad k = 0.433 \ psi \ per \ ft$$

$$H = \frac{psi}{k}$$

$$H = \frac{95}{.433}$$

$$H = 219.4 \ ft$$

90) We selected answer B because:

OSHA standard 1910.1000 is a performance standard that deals with more than one industry, which also makes it a horizontal standard.

91) We selected answer D because:

Accidents are usually multi-causal in nature and cannot be attributed entirely too any single factor.

92) We selected answer A because:

Progressive companies believe the proper way to deal with minor rule infractions is to issue an oral reprimand for the first offense. Progressive discipline is then administered for additional violations.

93) We selected answer C because:

Very toxic or poisonous gases do not require a safety relief device because of the hazard that release of these materials could cause. Most other bottled or compressed gases are required to be equipped with frangible disks, fusible disks, bursting discs, etc.

94) We selected answer C because:

Acclimatization to heat is generally achieved by having the employee exposed to the hot environment for two hours per day for one or two weeks.

95) We selected answer C because:

Should you choose to use "before and after testing" as an indicator of training effectiveness, the tests should cover the same areas but be phrased differently. This allows a determination to be made concerning comprehension levels, rather than "read and remember" skills.

96) We selected answer C because:

Accident investigation has as its primary purpose the prevention of similar occurrences and the discovery of hazards. The intent is not to place blame or administer discipline, but rather to determine how responsibilities may be defined or clarified and to reduce error producing situations. Accident investigation should improve the safety of operations, if accident investigation is used for punitive measures, the tool has the reverse effect.

97) We selected answer D because:

There are no universally agreed upon indirect costs of accidents within the health and safety community. Consequently, the term uninsured costs has grown in popularity because it has some standardization. However it is generally agreed that the indirect costs of accident include, but are not limited to:

- Cost of overtime for workers not injured
- Cost of training new worker to replace injured
- Cost of wages paid to accident investigators
- Cost of wages paid to unproductive workers due to accident
- Cost of damage to material and equipment
- Cost of medical not covered by insurance

98) We selected answer D because:

H.W. Heinrich in 1931 developed a theory of accident prevention, which was based on five axioms. One of which was the domino theory of accident causation. This theory modeled the accident sequence with five dominoes standing on end. As shown here, the dominoes represent the factors of ancestry or social environment, fault of the person, the unsafe act or condition, the accident and lastly, the injury. Once any one domino starts to fall there is nothing you can do to stop the sequence, however if you break the chain of dominoes by removing the center domino (unsafe act/condition), the accident sequence is aborted and an injury will not occur. Heinrich stated it this way:

" The occurrence of an injury invariably results from a completed sequence of factors the last one of these being the injury itself. The accident which caused the injury is in turn invariably caused or permitted directly by the unsafe act of a person and/or a mechanical or physical hazard."*

* Industrial Accident Prevention, 4th ed., McGraw-Hill Book Company, New York.

This accident causation model has largely been replaced by the more modern concept of multiple cause that envisions many factors combining to set the stage for accidental loss.

99) We selected answer D because:

According to the NSC, OJT or JIT is widely used because it allows the worker to produce during the training period. The primary instruction is the demonstration or demonstration-performance method of training.

100) We selected answer D because:

You are required by OSHA to post the citation at or near the location of the violation for three days or until corrected whichever is longer.

Self-Assessment Exam Four Questions

1) Within general industry, Lockout/Tagout programs only apply to electrical or high pressure utility systems.
   A) True.
   B) False.
   C) False, it only applies to electrical systems.
   D) True, unless OSHA-approved audits are performed annually.

2) Arrange the following hazard control steps in the proper sequence: (1) guard the hazard (2) engineer the hazard out if possible (3) educate personnel.
   A) 2,1,3.
   B) 3,1,2.
   C) 1,2,3.
   D) 3,2,1.

3) Which of the following is **not** a characteristic of local exhaust ventilation, when compared to dilution ventilation?
   A) Is more suitable for highly toxic substances.
   B) Is very good for ventilating point source emissions.
   C) Costs less than dilution ventilation.
   D) Uses less air than dilution ventilation.

4) The minimum amount of electric current passing through the body to produce a fatality is:
   A) 7 amps.
   B) 2 amps.
   C) 500-750 mA.
   D) 70-100 mA.

5) The mean plus two standard deviations, estimates what percentage of the distribution in a *normal* distribution?
   A) 95.5 %
   B) 98.5 %
   C) 85 %
   D) 50 %

6) The horizontal grouping of elements in the periodic table is called a

_____.
   A)   Tribe.
   B)   Period.
   C)   Group or Family.
   D)   Element.

7) The atomic number of an element indicates the total number of:
   A)   Neutrons.
   B)   Protons.
   C)   Protons and neutrons.
   D)   Electrons.

8) A temperature of 70 degrees F equals _____ degrees Rankin.
   A)   273 degrees.
   B)   530 degrees.
   C)   460 degrees.
   D)   203 degrees.

9) Which of the following is the **most correct** concerning the development and establishment of state plans under the provisions of the Federal OSHAct?
   A)   State plans must be as effective as the Federal program.
   B)   State plans are 100% funded for the first five years by the Federal program.
   C)   State CSHOs must have the same qualifications as their federal counterpart.
   D)   State plans do not have to have the same trade secret safeguards as the Federal program.

10) Which of the following agencies publishes standards and issues approvals for fire detection equipment?
   A)   MSHA-NIOSH.
   B)   ASTM-OSHA.
   C)   UL-NFPA.
   D)   NFPA-FM.

11) Which of the following is Public Law 91-596?
    A) Occupational Safety and Health Act.
    B) Federal Coal Mine Health and Safety Act.
    C) Federal Metal and Nonmetallic Mine Safety Act.
    D) Federal Mine Safety and Health Act.

12) Which of the following organizations issues the **most** standards in the U.S.?
    A) FM.
    B) UL.
    C) ANSI.
    D) NIOSH.

13) Which of the following two laws combine to form the Combined Gas Law?
    A) Boyle's and Charles' Laws.
    B) Dalton's and Newton's Laws.
    C) Pascal's and Charles' Laws.
    D) Adiabatic and Isothermal Laws.

14) Which of the following **best** describes the function of the Wilkes-Miran Analyzer?
    A) A general-purpose gas analyzer using IR detection techniques.
    B) A general-purpose hydrocarbon detector.
    C) A unique analyzer able to detect the presence of hydrocarbons in soils (used extensively in detecting storage tank leaks).
    D) A Combustible Gas Detector with an Oxygen sensor and alarm features.

15) ANSI standard Z 53.1 specifies which color to signify danger?
    A) Yellow.
    B) Yellow and Black stripes.
    C) Orange.
    D) Red.

16) The OSHA Permissible Exposure Limit (PEL) for asbestos fibers is an 8-hour TWA airborne concentration of 0.1 fibers per cubic centimeter of air as determined by the membrane filter method. What is the length of the fibers to be counted using this method?
    A) 3 micrometers.
    B) 5 micrometers.
    C) 8 micrometers.
    D) 7 micrometers.

17) In order to engender trust, OSHA's VPP approach to applicants is based on all the following principles **except?**
    A) The VPP is strictly voluntary.
    B) During the application process, prior to approval, the application is confidential.
    C) Under the OSH Act, compliance with the provisions of the Act and the standards set under the authority of the Act is mandatory.
    D) VPP participants will work independently to resolve any safety and health problems that may arise during participation.

18) The ASME *Boiler and Pressure Vessel Code* requires most pressure vessels to have safety devices (i.e. relief valves, fusible plugs, etc.) to adequately protect against overpressure, chemical reaction, or other abnormal conditions. When discharge lines are provided to carry discharge away from safety valves, the area of the discharge pipe should be _____ the area of the valve outlet(s)?
    A) Greater than.
    B) Less than.
    C) Equal to.
    D) Equal to or greater than.

19) 40CFR264 requires that the generators of hazardous waste must do all of the following **except?**

    A) Develop a written schedule for inspecting monitoring equipment, safety and emergency equipment, security devices and operating and structural equipment.

    B) Develop a contingency plan that describes the actions that facility personnel must take in case of fire, explosions or unplanned releases of hazardous waste.

    C) Make arrangements with the local fire, police and emergency teams to ensure their awareness and that they can respond within 10 minutes of notification.

    D) Develop a waste analysis plan that describes the details for analyzing each type of hazardous waste.

20) The eye contains all of the following **except?**

    A) Rods and Cones.

    B) Cochlea.

    C) Cornea.

    D) Retina.

21) Exposure to which of the following will **not** cause Pneumoconiosis?

    A) Lead.

    B) Asbestos.

    C) Coal dust.

    D) Quartz dust.

22) Which of the following fan laws is stated incorrectly?

    A) CFM varies indirectly as fan speed.

    B) SP varies as the square of fan speed.

    C) HP varies as the cube of the fan speed.

    D) TP varies as the square of fan speed.

23) In ventilation work, TP or Total Pressure is?

    A) The difference between SP and VP.

    B) Measured parallel to the axis of flow.

    C) Normally positive on the suction side.

    D) The product of SP and VP.

24) Which of the following sampling strategies is appropriate for determining if an exposure is above the ceiling concentration?
   A) Grab sampling.
   B) Dosimeters.
   C) 15 min personal monitoring.
   D) 8 hour personal monitoring.

25) Which of the following techniques would be used to determine the effectiveness of recently implemented controls to reduce the exposure to benzene?
   A) Draeger tubes and pumps in the work area.
   B) Blood tests every other week.
   C) Saliva test before work each shift.
   D) Urine test after the work shift.

26) In welding practice, the term *"GTAW"* represents which of the following?
   A) Gas Torch-Atomizing Welding.
   B) Gas Torch-Arc Waste.
   C) Gas Tungsten Arc-Welding.
   D) Gas Tungsten Atomizing-Welding.

27) Which of the following is known as the "Hazwoper" standard?
   A) OSHA 1926.120
   B) OSHA 1910.147
   C) OSHA 1910.120
   D) OSHA 1910.38

28) When respirator qualitative fit testing required by OSHA is conducted, which of the following is used to determine odor threshold?
   A) Isoamyl Acetate.
   B) Saccharin Solution.
   C) Isophorone.
   D) Sodium Acetate.

29) American National Standard Z89.1-1997 establishes specifications for helmets (hardhats) to protect the heads of industrial workers from impact and penetration by falling objects and from high-voltage electrical shock. Which of the following classes offers low voltage protection?

    A)   A.
    B)   C.
    C)   E.
    D)   G.

30) According to OSHA, at what depth must a trench be shored or cut to the angle of repose?

    A)   Greater than 4 feet.
    B)   5 feet or more.
    C)   4 feet.
    D)   6 feet or more.

31) According to OSHA, what spacing is required between the required ladders in excavations classified as trenches?

    A)   50 feet.
    B)   100 feet.
    C)   10 feet.
    D)   30 feet.

32) A test apparatus described as a drum half submerged in water, divided into chambers, with openings in the center and in each chamber would **most likely** be which of the following?

    A)   Dry Gas Meter.
    B)   Frictionless Piston Meter.
    C)   Wet test meter.
    D)   Mariotti bottle.

33) In performing ventilation measurements, the use of a pitot tube in the field is limited to flow rates above which of the following ranges?

    A)   400 - 600 fpm.
    B)   600 - 800 fpm.
    C)   800 - 1,000 fpm.
    D)   1,000 - 2,000 fpm.

34) What is the **most commonly** operated flow rate when using a Midget Impinger for particulate sampling?
    A) 2.8 L/min.
    B) L/min.
    C) 10 L/min.
    D) 15 L/min.

35) Which of the following is **not** an acceptable guarding procedure for a part-revolution clutch power press?
    A) Die enclosure guard.
    B) Reduction of timing to 25 cycles per minute.
    C) Pullback restraint guards.
    D) Adjustable barrier guards.

36) The OSHA Permissible Exposure Limit (PEL) for coal tar pitch volatiles is 0.2 mg/m^3. Which of the following would **not** be considered coal tar pitch volatiles under this standard?
    A) Asphalt.
    B) Acridine.
    C) Chrysene.
    D) Anthracene.

37) American National Standard Z89.1-1997 establishes specifications for helmets (hardhats) to protect the heads of industrial workers from impact and penetration by falling objects and from high-voltage electrical shock. Which of the following classes offers high voltage protection?
    A) A.
    B) C.
    C) E.
    D) G.

38) Which of the following analytical methods would **most likely** be used in the sampling for Toluene, Xylene, Hexane and Benzene?
    A) Ion chromatography.
    B) Visible spectrophotometry.
    C) Gas chromatography with flame ionization.
    D) Gravimetric methods.

39) The Mine Safety and Health Administration (MSHA) requires certain training for each new underground miner. Which of the following **best** describes that training?
    A)   Performance based training.
    B)   Specification based training.
    C)   180 hours of on-the-job training.
    D)   10 hours of classroom education.

40) Which article of the National Electrical Code deals with hazardous locations?
    A)   Article 407.
    B)   Article 101.
    C)   Article 20.
    D)   Article 500.

41) Which of the following ANSI Standards deals with accident reporting?
    A)   ANSI Z16.1
    B)   ANSI A17.1
    C)   ANSI Z87.1
    D)   ANSI Z89.1

42) If a storage facility is used to store flammable products, where the possibility of explosion if involved in a fire was high, what would be the maximum travel distance to exits, with and without a fire sprinkler system installed, allowed by NFPA 101®, *Life Safety Code*®?
    A)   75 feet without and 150 feet with an approved fire sprinkler system.
    B)   100 feet without and 150 feet with an approved fire sprinkler system.
    C)   200 feet without and 200 feet with an approved fire sprinkler system.
    D)   75 feet without and 100 feet with an approved fire sprinkler system.

43) A gas mask is to be used for protection against Hydrochloric Acid. What color should the canister be?
    A)   Blue.
    B)   Black.
    C)   Yellow.
    D)   Green.

44) When performing a pitot tube traverse of a round duct in a ventilation system, it is advisable to measure in two planes perpendicular to each other. What is the number of measurements per plane?
   A) 5.
   B) 10.
   C) 20.
   D) 30.

45) When performing WBGT measurements, the use of a globe thermometer is required. How long should the globe thermometer be in place before reliable readings can be obtained?
   A) 1 hour.
   B) 30 minutes.
   C) 20 minutes.
   D) 5 minutes.

46) What is the first step when doing CPR?
   A) Check airway.
   B) Check breathing.
   C) Check circulation.
   D) Start chest thrusts.

47) The inverse square law as applied to illumination states:
   A) The light source as perceived varies inversely as the square of the power.
   B) The light intensity of the source varies inversely as the distance in lumens.
   C) Light intensity on a surface varies inversely with the square of the distance between the source and the surface.
   D) Surface illumination varies directly with the inverse square of the distance.

48) According to 29 CFR 1910.23, a standard railing shall consist of top rail, intermediate rail, and posts, and shall have a vertical height of ___ inches nominal from upper surface of top rail to floor, platform, runway, or ramp level.
   A) 36.
   B) 40.
   C) 42.
   D) 48.

49) According to 1910.145, which of the following is incorrect when posting a Danger tag?

    A) The signal word shall be readable at a minimum distance of 7 feet or greater.

    B) The message shall be presented in text or pictographs or both.

    C) The tags shall be affixed as close as possible to the hazard.

    D) Employees must be informed as to the meaning of the signs.

50) Which of the following field instruments would be used to measure air velocity in the opening of a paint spray booth?

    A) Rotating Vane Anemometer.

    B) Velometer.

    C) Smoke tube.

    D) Pitot tube.

51) If you have tested two sets of data and there is no statistical difference between the data sets, then you are said to have perfect?

    A) Lack of variance.

    B) Statistical significance.

    C) Coefficient.

    D) Correlation.

52) Your company hires a worker unaware of his existing back problem. Three weeks later, this person aggravates his back problem while on the job. Workers compensation would:

    A) Deny the claim based on ADA.

    B) Pay 100% for a new injury.

    C) Pay only medical expenses and prescriptions.

    D) Deny the claim based on an existing condition.

53) Untrained personnel who are unfamiliar with the product or the hazards involved but who want to help in an emergency is a reason why the latches on the outside of aircraft to release cockpit canopies are marked. Which of the following is **not** true about such devices?

    A) Such devices must be foolproof in an emergency.
    B) They require little physical effort to operate.
    C) They can be easy to operate when only a few words of instruction are provided.
    D) They must be labeled in multiple languages.

54) What types of ladders are approved for electrical work?

    A) Metal.
    B) Only wooden ladders.
    C) Nonconductive ladders, including wooden.
    D) Ladders are not approved for electrical work.

55) A transport truck has been involved in an accident. The truck is overturned and the driver has been overcome and has a cherry red skin color. The air smells of bitter almond. Which of the following chemicals would you **most suspect** of being transported in the overturned truck?

    A) Chlorobenzene (C_6H_5Cl).
    B) Furfural (C_4H_3OCHO).
    C) Hydrogen Cyanide (HCN).
    D) Hydrogen Sulfide (H_2S).

56) One method of controlling noise is by the use of enclosures. Enclosures are designed to:

    A) Isolate the individual from the noise source.
    B) Reduce the noise level at the source.
    C) Reduce the internal sound pressure build up.
    D) Increase the distance between the source and the receiver.

57) The primary reason safety professionals perform accident investigation is to determine causal conditions. The responsibility for implementing corrective actions is **best** placed with the:

    A)   Supervisor.
    B)   Safety Administrator.
    C)   Senior Safety Engineer.
    D)   Plant Manager.

58) All of the following are valid reasons for accident (mishap) investigation **except?**

    A)   Prevent reoccurrence of similar events.
    B)   Establish casual factors.
    C)   Provide vehicle for discipline.
    D)   Provide data for trend analysis.

59) If an employee owns her own PPE, who is responsible to ensure it is maintained?

    A)   Employee.
    B)   Employer.
    C)   Union Rep.
    D)   Supervisor.

60) Who has the approval authority for Safety Gas Cans?

    A)   DOT.
    B)   OSHA.
    C)   UL.
    D)   DOT.

61) You are responding to a silo where one person has entered and is now presumed dead. Which of the following instruments would you take with you?

    A)   CGI with Oxygen sensor.
    B)   IR Spectrometer.
    C)   GCMS.
    D)   Pitot Tube.

62) Which of the following would be classified a Class "A" fire?
    A) A Fire involving ordinary combustibles.
    B) A Fire involving flammable liquids.
    C) A Fire involving combustible metals.
    D) A Fire involving live electrical equipment.

63) When developing an emergency plan, the first step should be to?
    A) Identify and evaluate the potential disasters.
    B) Assess the potential harm that may be caused.
    C) Evaluate how many company assets are required.
    D) Decide on the chain of command.

64) What is the **primary** consideration when preparing for a potential disaster?
    A) Selecting the emergency committee.
    B) Identifying a person to be the on-scene commander.
    C) Doing advanced emergency planning.
    D) Having a list of State and Federal directives that you may need.

65) Under the provisions of the Resource Conservation and Recovery Act (RCRA), generators of hazardous waste have the responsibility to prepare a Uniform Hazardous Waste Manifest which is a transport and control device that stays with the hazardous waste at all times. RCRA also requires generators to maintain copies of the manifest for a period of?

    A) Five years.
    B) Only until delivered and signed for at a TSD.
    C) Three years.
    D) Thirty years.

66) Many small businesses produce hazardous waste that is regulated by the Resource Conservation and Recovery Act (RCRA). If regulated, EPA will control this hazardous waste from the moment it is generated until its ultimate disposal. Which of the following businesses would be considered a small quantity generator by the EPA?

    A) You produce more than _____ and less than _____ pounds of hazardous waste in a calendar month.

    B) 200 and 2,000.

    C) 220 and 2,200.

    D) 400 and 4,000.

    E) 440 and 4,400.

67) All of the following are required steps to perform chain-of-custody on evidence collected during an accident investigation **except?**

    A) Collect.

    B) Track.

    C) Identify.

    D) Log movement.

68) What type of fire extinguishing equipment is required for welding operations?

    A) Class A.

    B) Class B.

    C) Class C.

    D) Suitable fire extinguishing equipment.

69) What type of eye protection is required for other workers exposed to welding operations or individuals observing welding operations?

    A) Safety glasses.

    B) Goggles with filters.

    C) Flame proof screens or goggles.

    D) No protections required.

70) Which of the following is a term used to describe the condition "epicondylitis"?
    A) Trigger finger.
    B) Rotator cuff.
    C) Roofer's wrist.
    D) Carpenter's elbow.

71) Who provides the required placards when shipping hazardous material?
    A) The driver.
    B) The carrier.
    C) The shipper.
    D) The manufacturer.

72) A hazardous material incident is a situation in which a hazardous material is or may be released into the environment. What is the first step when responding to an incident?
    A) Control.
    B) Evaluation.
    C) Safety.
    D) Recognition.

73) All of the following concerning flammable inside storage areas are true **except?** Inside storage locations must be provided with:
    A) A clear aisle at least 22 inches wide.
    B) A raised 4 inch sill.
    C) Self-closing fire doors.
    D) Either gravity or mechanical exhaust system.

74) Which of the following lists the three distinct parts of a "means of egress"?
    A) Exit access, exit, and exit discharge.
    B) Door, passageway, and ramps.
    C) Door opening device, door, and exit light.
    D) Horizontal exits, stairs, and ramps.

75) A Commercial Motor Vehicle transporting hazardous materials is required to display placards in which of the following locations?

    A) Front, rear and both sides of vehicle.
    B) Front, rear and both sides of hazmat container.
    C) Front, rear, top and both sides of vehicle.
    D) Front, rear, top and both sides of hazmat container.

76) When experiencing a natural emergency, emergency preparedness plans usually call for which of the following as the first consideration?

    A) Turn the responsibility over to the authorities for protection of resources.
    B) Safeguard people and abandon systems.
    C) Shutdown processes involving hazardous/toxic materials.
    D) Safeguard both personnel and equipment/processes.

77) A door latch assembly, incorporating a device that releases the latch upon application of a force in the direction of exit travel, is the definition of?

    A) Door knob.
    B) Panic hardware.
    C) Secure door guard.
    D) Emergency protection hardware.

78) If you have an emergency response situation and need to set up a command center, always set it up in the:

    A) Cold zone.
    B) Warm zone.
    C) Hot zone.
    D) Outside of all zones.

79) Which of the following is the **best** demonstration for auditor impartiality during an audit?

    A) By being expertly prepared to conduct the audit.
    B) By holding an accredited third-party professional certification.
    C) By signing a statement confirming impartiality and will report objectively all on the audit.
    D) By being free from any line or operational responsibility for the activity being audited.

80) When auditing a company's conformance with ISO 14001 and OHSAS 18001 management systems, which of the following **best** provides minimally acceptable verification that the company is reviewing proposed or new legal requirements for applicability to the organization?
   A) A document identifying the date of any review of new or proposed legal requirements and a statement determining applicability.
   B) A certified letter from an attorney stating that the company complies with all legal requirements.
   C) An e-mail from a legal update review service demonstrating that new legal requirements are routinely transmitted to the company.
   D) A signed consultant's report outlining the legal requirements applicable to the organization.

81) Which of the following **best** describes the use of the Critical Incident Technique method during an incident investigation?
   A) A method to identify mechanical integrity issues in chemical process equipment.
   B) An open-ended retrospective method of interviews that identify the critical aspects of an incident.
   C) A guided discussion as part of pre-emergency planning exercise.
   D) A sampling of human behaviors through observation.

82) Which of the following is **not** considered a basic principle of loss control?
   A) "An unsafe act, an unsafe condition, and an accident are all symptoms of something wrong in the management system."
   B) "We can predict that certain sets of circumstances will produce severe injuries. These circumstances can be identified and controlled."
   C) "The key to effective line safety performance is management procedures that fix accountability."
   D) "Safety must be managed as a special company function - set apart from the normal planning process to ensure management's commitment to safety is clearly visible among employees."

83) The OHSAS 18001 specification requires only minimal documentation. It is important that documented OH&S procedures are developed and adequately controlled. A compilation of documents that form the basis for the management system is normally called?
   A) List of Documents.
   B) Safety Policy Manual.
   C) Master List.
   D) Document Inventory Index.

84) A safety director who normally works in an advisory capacity has been told that if she detects any imminent hazards of specified types, she, may immediately and independently shut down the operation involved. The directive is in writing and comes from the vice president for manufacturing. This represents what type of authority?
   A) Undelegated authority.
   B) Staff authority.
   C) Informal authority.
   D) Functional authority.

85) The scope of the ISO 19011 standard is to provide guidance on the principles of:
   A) Managing and conducting an occupational health and safety system audit.
   B) Managing and implementing an environmental management system.
   C) Managing and implementing an occupational health and safety management system.
   D) Managing and conducting quality and environmental management system audits.

86) The U.S. Voluntary Protection Programs (VPP) as administered by Occupational Safety and Health Administration is an optional safety-related management system. The four components associated with participating in the VPP include a management commitment, one or more work site analyses, hazard prevention and control, and establishing:
   A) Program goals and objectives.
   B) A joint labor-management committee.
   C) Safety and health training.
   D) A written safety policy.

87) In choosing an appropriate organizational model, a manager should understand that:
   A) The best arrangement reduces the manager's span of control to the minimum number of supervised persons to ensure that supervision is maintained as closely as possible.
   B) A staff unit assists line managers with the burdens of broad supervisory responsibilities.
   C) There are multiple arrangements that will produce the best results with minimum difficulty in the situation in which the organization operates.
   D) The best arrangement reduces the number of organizational layers as much as possible so that the communication lines between the manager and the subordinates will be short.

88) Periodic evaluations of employee performance are **most valuable** if the ratings of each employee are:
   A) Based principally on his or her personality traits.
   B) Stringent, containing criticisms as well as praise.
   C) Based entirely on factors that can be measured objectively.
   D) Discussed with him or her and directions for improvement indicated.

89) Which should a safety professional recommend to line management when significant process or operational changes are being considered?
   A) Performing comprehensive, change analyses during the decision-making process.
   B) Ensuring all recommendations from root cause analyses have been implemented.
   C) Obtaining buy-in from all employees of the benefits related to the process changes.
   D) Obtaining buy-in from regulators of the process changes.

90) ANSI Z16.2 "Method of recording basic facts relating to the nature and occurrence of work injuries" contains an analytical category of accident that identifies the object, substance, or premises that contained a hazardous condition. This category is called?

    A) Hazard index.
    B) Agency of Accident.
    C) Hazardous Condition.
    D) Accident Classification.

91) On the OSHA 300 Log, all the following are classified as injuries **except?**

    A) Electrocution.
    B) Pharyngitis.
    C) Chipped tooth.
    D) Amputation.

Five year mishap history in a manufacturing facility

Year	Total Recordable Injury and Illness	Lost Work Days	Lost Work Day Cases	Days Away from Work	Days of Restricted Work Activity	Hours
1	92	1932	67	1565	367	1,398,765
2	88	2002	81	1622	380	1,456,732
3	119	1821	98	1384	137	1,129,565
4	118	1754	90	1316	438	1,623,451
5	122	1234	98	740	494	1,834,225

92) Determine the cumulative DART accident rate for the 5 years shown in the chart.

    A) 27.7
    B) 2.76
    C) 10.9
    D) 11.7

93) An employee at your plant strained her wrist. The plant RN had the employee use an elastic wristlet until the wrist had healed. How would this be recorded on the OSHA 300 Log?
   A) All other illnesses.
   B) Skin Disorder.
   C) Injury.
   D) Not recordable.

94) Examples of indirect costs of an incident include:
   A) Drug testing and ambulance service.
   B) Incident review and process delays.
   C) Medical treatment supplies and medical related treatment.
   D) Job accommodations and new equipment.

95) A reading of 1 percent carbon dioxide in air is equal to how many parts per million (ppm)?
   A) 50 ppm.
   B) 1000 ppm.
   C) 10,000 ppm.
   D) 100,000 ppm.

96) Throughout accident investigations, the interviewing of witnesses is often required to determine facts relative to the event. Which of the following choices offers the **best** place to conduct interviews for safety investigations?
   A) In a secure board room equipped with sound recording devices.
   B) Privately in a conference room.
   C) At the employees' work area.
   D) In your office with door shut.

97) Sampling often involves the use of filters to collect particulates. Standard filters are 37 mm in diameter and are usually placed in a closed-face cassette with a backup pad to avoid contamination. The OSHA Asbestos Standard is an exception and requires which of the following:
   A) A larger 47 mm filter.
   B) A smaller open-face cassette.
   C) A glass fiber filter.
   D) A 20 mm cyclone with a preweighed filter.

98) There are four major sections of the Emergency Response Guidebook that provide identification and emergency response actions. The four color-coded sections are as follows:
   A) Yellow, blue, orange, green.
   B) Orange, green, yellow, red.
   C) Red, green, yellow, white.
   D) Red, green, yellow, blue.

99) A single pump is used to supply hydraulic pressure to a door closer in a regulated biohazard area. The door is closed remotely if an accident should occur. The facility maintenance/engineering staff was concerned about the high probability of failure. The old pump (1×10^{-8}) was replaced with a new dual pump arrangement. With the new dual pump arrangement, either pump can supply enough hydraulic pressure to close the door. Additionally, each pump is a different type and has different probabilities of failure. Pump "A" has a probability of failure of 1×10^{-4} and pump "B" has a failure rate of 1×10^{-3}. Which of the following statements **best** describes this situation?
   A) Maintenance/engineering should be commended for a good job.
   B) The success of this important safety system has been improved considerably.
   C) The failure rate has increased by a factor of 10.
   D) The failure rate has decreased by a factor of 20.

100) The mean plus two standard deviations, estimates what percentage of the distribution in a *normal* distribution?
   A) 95 %
   B) 99 %
   C) 68 %
   D) 50 %

Self-Assessment Exam Four Answers

1)   We selected answer B because:

At one time, Lockout/Tagout was only widely applied to electrical systems. However, for some time it has also applied to any mechanical system, which possesses potential energy, which could be released accidentally thus causing injury. The key is to make sure that all energy is a zero and will remain that way until restarted.

2)   We selected answer A because:

Engineering is always the first and most successful method of dealing with a problem. Second choice would be to guard the hazard, and last to educate the human element. Some safety texts break down "guarding the hazard" into (1) incorporation of safety devices and (2) providing warning devices. Guarding the hazard is also classified as administrative controls. "Educating personnel" may also be sub-divided into (1) developing and implementing operating procedures and employee training programs and (2) using personal protective equipment. Providing hand washing facilities would be considered an administrative control.

3)   We selected answer C because:

Local exhaust ventilation almost always costs more than dilution ventilation. Dilution ventilation is defined as the removing or adding of air to keep the concentration of a contaminant below hazardous levels. The process can use natural or forced air movement through open doors, windows, etc. or, exhaust fans can be mounted on roofs, walls, or windows. Local exhaust systems trap the air contaminant near its source which usually makes this method much more effective, but more expensive than dilution. Exhaust Ventilation can be used to remove flammable vapors, mists or powders to a safe location and to confine and control combustible residues.

4) We selected answer D because:

The range of 70-100 mA is widely accepted as enough current to produce a fatality. Many cases of deaths from low voltages have been reported.

5) We selected answer A because:

The mean plus two standard deviations will estimate the point at which 95.5% of the observations will fall.

6) We selected answer B because:

Vertical groupings are families and horizontal groupings are periods.

7) We selected answer B because:

The Atomic number of a substance refers to the total number of protons in the nucleus.

8) We selected answer B because:

To convert t_f to t_R you must add 460

$$70 + 460 = 530$$

9) We selected answer A because:

OSHA requires that state plans provide an overall program at least as effective as the Federal program and may include areas not covered by the Federal standard. The indicators of effectiveness are listed at 1902.4.

10) We selected answer C because:

The National Fire Protection Association publishes several standards on fire detection and alarm systems, UL issues approvals for these and other types of signaling equipment.

11) We selected answer A because:

Public Law 91-596, is the Occupational Safety and Health Act. Public Law 91-173, December 30, 1969, was the Federal Coal Mine Health and Safety Act. Public Law 91-577, is the Federal Metal and Non-metallic Mine Safety Act. Public Law 91-173, November 9, 1977, is the Federal Mine Safety and Health Act.

The General Duty clause is part of Public Law 91-596 that says "Each employer shall furnish to each of his employees employment and a place of employment which are free from recognized hazards that are causing or likely to cause death or serious physical harm to his employees".

12) We selected answer C because:

The largest standard setting organization in the United States is the American National Standards Institute, which currently has over 3,000 standards dealing with an extremely wide variety of subjects.

13) We selected answer A because:

In solving true gas problems Boyle's and Charles' laws may be combined. The gas law is expressed:

$$\frac{P_1 V_1}{T_1} = \frac{P_2 V_2}{T_2}$$

14) We selected answer A because:

The Wilkes-Miran Gas Analyzers are used to detect any gas, which absorbs infrared radiation in wavelengths between 2.5 and 14.5 μm. Most gases can be measured over a sensitivity range of less than 1 ppm up to several percent.

15) We selected answer D because:

The American National Standards Institute (ANSI) standard Z53.1

"Safety Color Coding for Marking Physical Hazards" denoted red as the color for danger, fire-protection equipment and for emergency stop switches. Yellow with or without black stripes is used for hazards and hazardous material storage cabinets. Orange is used to mark dangerous parts of machinery and or equipment.

16) We selected answer B because:

Permissible Exposure Limit (PEL) for asbestos is 0.1 fiber per cubic centimeter of air as an eight-hour time-weighted average (TWA), with an excursion limit (EL) of 1.0 asbestos fibers per cubic centimeter over a 30-minute period. The employer must ensure that no one is exposed above these limits. A fiber is particle that is 5 microns (um) or longer, with a length-to-width ratio of 3 to 1 or longer. The ratio of the length of a fiber to its diameter (e.g. 3:1, 5:1 aspect ratios).

Matrix:
OSHA Permissible Exposure Limits:
Time Weighted Average......................... 0.1 fiber/cc
Excursion Level (30 minutes)................. 1.0 fiber/cc

Collection Procedure:
A known volume of air is drawn through a 25-mm diameter cassette containing a mixed-cellulose ester filter. The cassette must be equipped with an electrically conductive 50-mm extension cowl. The sampling time and rate are chosen to give a fiber density of between 100 to 1,300 fibers/mm(2) on the filter.

Recommended Sampling Rate....................... 0.5 to 5.0 liters/minute (L/min)
Recommended Air Volumes:
Minimum...................................... 25 L
Maximum...................................... 2,400 L

17) We selected answer D because:

According to the **VPP Philosophy,** the VPP approach to applicants is based on the following principles:

- Voluntarism
- Confidentiality
- Compliance and Beyond
- Hazard Prevention
- Cooperation - VPP staff and approved VPP participants will work together to resolve any safety and health problems that may arise during participation.

The program consists of four major elements, management commitment, work site analysis, hazard prevention & control and safety & health training.

Injury and Illness History Requirements. Injury and illness history at the site is evaluated using a 3-year total case incident rate (TCIR) and a 3-year day away, restricted, and/or transfer case incident rate (DART rate). (See Appendix A.) The 3-year TCIR and DART rates must be compared to the most recently published Bureau of Labor Statistics (BLS) national average for the three or four-digit (if available) Standard Industrial Classification code (SIC). The TCIR and DART rates must be compared to the five- or six-digit North American Industrial Classification System (NAICS) code for the industry in which the applicant is classified when the NAICS system is adopted. The BLS publishes SIC and NAICS industry averages 2 years after data is collected. (For example, in calendar year 2003, calendar year 2001 national averages will be available and used for comparison). Both the 3-year TCIR and the 3-year DART rate must be below the most recently published BLS national average for the specific SIC or NAICS code. The requirement for a Star sight to have a 3-year injury and illness rate that is below their respective industry is to be modified such that an applicant/participant's rate must be below their respective industries injury and illness rate plus 10%.

As a result a Star worksite may have an injury and illness rate above the national average if it is within 10% of that BLS average.

18)   We selected answer D because:

According to ASME B31 series, *Pressure Piping*, sectional areas of a discharge pipe shall not be less than the full area of the valve outlets discharging there into and the discharge pipe shall be as short as possible and so arranged as to avoid undue stresses on the valve or valves. It is recommended that individual discharge lines be used for each valve, but if two or more valves are combined, the discharge piping shall be designed with sufficient flow area to prevent blowout of steam or other fluids.

19) We selected answer C because:

According to 40CFR264 –

Sec. 264.37 Arrangements with local authorities.

(a) The owner or operator must attempt to make the following arrangements, as appropriate for the type of waste handled at his facility and the potential need for the services of these organizations:

(1) Arrangements to familiarize police, fire departments, and emergency response teams with the layout of the facility, properties of hazardous waste handled at the facility and associated hazards, places where facility personnel would normally be working, entrances to and roads inside the facility, and possible evacuation routes;

<u>No time or distance constraints listed.</u>

Sec. 264.15 General inspection requirements.

(a) The owner or operator must inspect his facility for malfunctions and deterioration, operator errors, and discharges which may be causing--or may lead to--(1) release of hazardous waste constituents to the environment or (2) a threat to human health. The owner or operator must conduct these inspections often enough to identify problems in time to correct them before they harm human health or the environment.

(b)(1) The owner or operator must develop and follow a written schedule for inspecting monitoring equipment, safety and emergency equipment, security devices, and operating and structural equipment (such as dikes and sump pumps) that are important to preventing, detecting, or responding to environmental or human health hazards.

Sec. 264.52 Content of contingency plan.

(a) The contingency plan must describe the actions facility personnel must take to comply with Secs. 264.51 and 264.56 in response to fires, explosions, or any unplanned sudden or non-sudden release of hazardous waste or hazardous waste constituents to air, soil, or surface water at the facility.

Sec. 264.13 General waste analysis.

(a)(1) Before an owner or operator treats, stores, or disposes of any hazardous wastes, or nonhazardous wastes if applicable under Sec. 264.113(d), he must obtain a detailed chemical and physical analysis of a representative sample of the wastes. At a minimum, the analysis must contain all the information which must be known to treat, store, or dispose of the waste in accordance with this part and part 268 of this chapter.

(b) The owner or operator must develop and follow a written waste analysis plan which describes the procedures which he will carry out to comply with paragraph (a) of this section. He must keep this plan at the facility. Doing proper maintenance, and sanitation of such equipment.

20) We selected answer B because:

The cochlea is a cone shaped winding structure in the inner ear containing the organ of corti, which is the receptor for hearing.

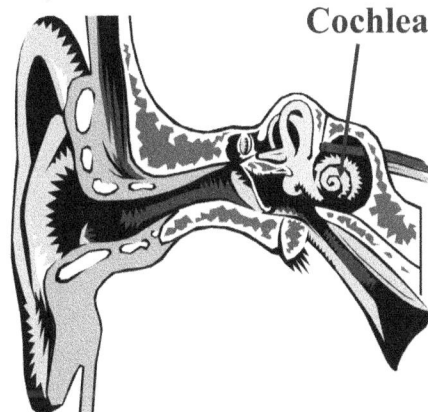

Cochlea

21) We selected answer A because:

Pneumoconiosis is called dusty lung and is any lung disease caused by the inhalation of substantial amounts of *particulate* matter in the lung.

22) We selected answer A because:

The laws governing fan operation provide the OHST with some very useful tools for dealing with ventilation problems where a change in capacity is required. The fan laws are:

- CFM varies **directly** as Fan Speed
- TP and SP varies as the square of the fan speed
- HP varies as the cube of the fan speed

23)   We selected answer B because:

Total Pressure is measured parallel to the direction of flow.

24)   We selected answer C because:

In industrial hygiene practice if instantaneous monitoring is not feasible, then the TLV-C can be assessed by sampling over a 15 minute period except for those substances which may cause immediate irritation when exposures are short.

25)   We selected answer D because:

Biological monitoring to determine the effectiveness of recent changes would involve urine tests to determine S-Phenylmercapturic or t,t-Muconic acid content after each work shift.

26)   We selected answer C because:

GTAW stands for Gas Tungsten Arc-Welding, which is a process that joins metals by heating them with an arc between a tungsten electrode and the work, shielding is obtained from a gas mixture. The process is often called TIG welding. Because of the inherent safety and health hazards involved in the welding process the OHST examination has historically contained several questions on the different processes and the hazards associated with each.

27)   We selected answer C because:

OSHA 1910.120 is known by the acronym "Hazwoper" which stands for HAZARDOUS WASTE OPERATIONS AND EMERGENCY RESPONSE STANDARD. There is no OSHA 1926.120. OSHA 1910.147 is the *Control of Hazardous Energy Standard*. OSHA 1910.38 is the *Employee Emergency Plans and Fire Prevention Plans Standard*.

28) We selected answer A because:

OSHA appendix "D" to section 1910.1025 "Qualitative fit test protocols" requires that during odor threshold testing three mason jars be filled with water. One cc of pure *Isoamyl Acetate* is added to one jar. Test subjects are then asked to identify which jar smells like banana oil.

Prior to respirator fitting, the individual must complete a federal OSHA Respiratory Medical Evaluation Questionnaire and the questionnaire must be reviewed by a licensed health care professional.

29) We selected answer D because:

Hard hats that are considered to be "OSHA approved" meet the minimum criteria established by the American National Standards (ANSI) and the International Safety Equipment Association (ISEA), in accordance with the most current ANSI/ISEA Z89.1-2009 standard. Hard hat impact protection is divided into two categories: Type I and Type II.

Type I Hard Hats are intended to reduce the force of impact resulting from a blow only to the top of the head. This form of impact, for example, may result from a hammer or nail gun falling from above.

Type II Hard Hats are intended to reduce the force of lateral impact resulting from a blow which may be received off-center, from the side, or to the top of the head. This form of impact, for example, may result from contact with the sharp corner of a side beam.

According to ANSI/ISEA Z89.1-2009 and Canadian CSA Z94.1-2005 standards, hard hat electrical performance is divided into three categories: Class E, Electrical; Class G, General, and; Class C, Conductive

Class E (Electrical) helmets intended to reduce the danger of exposure to high voltage electrical conductors, proof tested at 20,000 volts. Class E is tested for force transmission first, then tested at 20,000 volts for 3 minutes, with 9 milliamps maximum current leakage; then tested at 30,000 volts, with no burn-through permitted.(formerly Class B)

Class G (General) helmets intended to reduce the danger of exposure to low voltage electrical conductors, proof tested at 2,200 volts. Class G is tested at 2,200 volts for 1 minute, with 3 milliamps max. leakage.

(formerly Class A)

Class C (Conductive) helmets not intended to provide protection from electrical conductors. Class C is not tested for electrical resistance. (no change in class designation)

30)   We selected answer B because:

Excavations that are less than 5 feet in depth do not require shoring or sloping, if examination of the ground is conducted by a competent person, who finds no indication of a potential cave-in. The "angle of repose" is the angle at which soil will no longer slide, in this instance it means to slope to a flat enough angle to prevent the soil from sliding back into the ditch. A quick review of OSHA 1926.651 and 652 is in order prior to taking the OHST examination.

31)   We selected answer A because:

Means of egress from trench excavations such as a stairway, ladder, ramp or other safe means of egress are required in trench excavations that are 4 feet or more in depth and located so as to require **no more than 25 feet of lateral travel** for workers. Ladders placed every 50 running feet of trench would provide a maximum of 25 feet of travel in each direction, assuming a initial ladder at the start of the trench run. OSHA 1926.651.

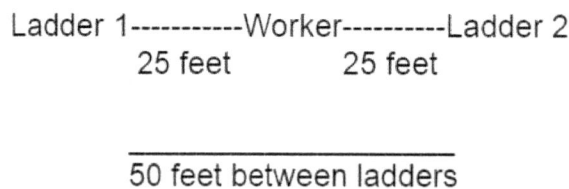

Ladder 1-----------Worker----------Ladder 2
            25 feet   25 feet

50 feet between ladders

32)   We selected answer C because:

The question accurately describes a wet test meter. The wet test meter is considered a secondary calibration standard. Other secondary standards are the dry-gas meter, and precision rotameter.

33) We selected answer B because:

Pitot tubes are generally limited in field use to velocities above 600 to 800 fpm because of the inaccuracy in reading the manometer. In the 600-800 fpm range the error is about 15%.

34) We selected answer A because:

Midget impingers are most commonly operated at 0.1 CFM or 2.8 L/min.

35) We selected answer B because:

Reduction of timing is not considered an acceptable guard against accidental activation or inadvertent placement of body parts within the hazard zone of power presses. On part-revolution presses guards must be:

- physical guards such as barrier guards
- protection devices such as restraints, pullbacks, two-hand controls or interlocked movable barriers

36) We selected answer A because:

OSHA currently defines coal tar pitch volatiles as the fused polycyclic hydrocarbons that volatilize from the distillation residues of coal, petroleum, wood, and other organic matter such as anthracene, benzo (a) pyrene (BaP), phenanthrene, acridine, chrysene, pyrene, etc. Asphalt is not included under the OSHA standard for coal tar pitch volatiles.

37) We selected answer C because:

Helmet Types

Class E (Electrical) helmets intended to reduce the danger of exposure to high voltage electrical conductors, proof tested at 20,000 volts.

Class G (General) helmets intended to reduce the danger of exposure to low voltage electrical conductors, proof tested at 2,200 volts.

Class C (Conductive) helmets not intended to provide protection from electrical conductors. Class C is not tested for electrical resistance. (no change in class designation)

Definitions expanded; new test protocol section, including preparation, mounting, number, and sequence of test samples; summary of failure criteria.

- Product tested within 3 inch circle on top of helmet in "as worn" position
- 2.2 pound pointed steel penetrator, with 60° angle, dropped from a simulated free-fall height of 8 feet
- Penetrator can't make contact w/ head form
- Test apparatus includes electronic contact indicator, velocity indicator, & electronic recording equipment
- No differentiation for helmet classes

38)   We selected answer C because:

Gas chromatography with flame ionization detection is the recommended analytical method to be used on all these hydrocarbons.

39)   We selected answer B because:

Throughout the history of The Mine Safety and Health Administration (MSHA) the organization has stressed the importance of training for miners. The training is expressly prescribed, "Every new underground miner shall receive no less than 40 hours of prescribed training". MSHA then lists the prescribed training complete with format. This is in contrast to the performance based training required by recent legislation, eg: the OSHA Hazard Communication Standard or the permit-required confined space standard.

40)   We selected answer D because:

Article 500 of the NEC deals with classifications of hazardous locations.

41) We selected answer A because:

ANSI Z16.1 "Method of Recording and Measuring Work Injury Experience." ANSI A17.1 "Elevators, Escalators, and Moving Walks." ANSI Z87.1 "Practice for Occupational and Educational Eye and Face Protection." ANSI Z89.1 "Protective Headware for Industrial Workers."

42) We selected answer D because:

Section 29 of the NFPA 101®, *Life Safety Code*®, provides guidance on the maximum travel distance to exits. If the hazard of the contents is classified as ordinary hazard, the distance to an exit could not exceed 200 feet, or 400 feet if equipped with an approved automatic fire sprinkler system. However, any area used for the storage of high hazard materials shall have an exit within 75 feet of the point where persons might be present. This distance can be extended to 100 feet when fire sprinkler protection is provided. Travel distances vary with different occupancies, again a review of the *Life Safety Code*® is certainly in order prior to the examination.

According to 29 CFR 1926, for fire control of flammable or combustible liquids, at least one portable fire extinguisher having a rating of not less than 20-B shall be located not less than 25 feet nor more than 75 feet from any storage area located outside.

43) We selected answer C because:

CONTAMINANT	COLOR
Ammonia Gas	Green
Organic Vapors	Black
Carbon Monoxide Gas	Blue
Acid Gas and Organic Vapors	Yellow

44) We selected answer B because:

Normally, when performing a pitot tube traverse of a round duct a minimum of 10 measurements per plane (20 per duct) are required. However, a smaller or larger number may be appropriate depending on the diameter of the duct. The following table illustrates one recommendation:

Diameter in Inches	Number of Measurements per Traverse
3 to 6	6
6 to 24	10
Larger than 24	20

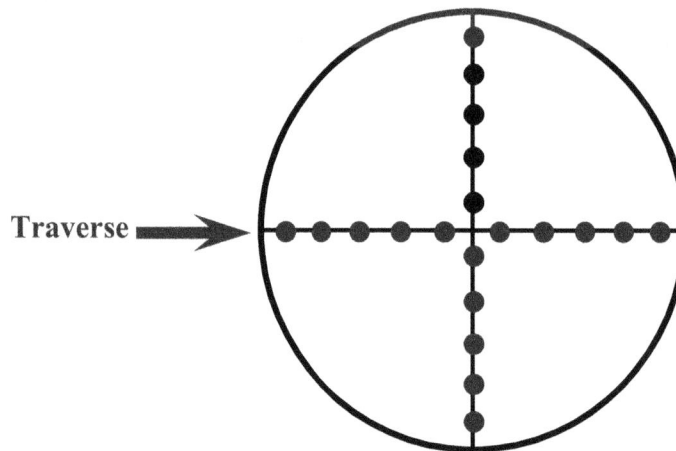

45) We selected answer C because:

The globe thermometer is a thin walled, blackened copper sphere 6 inches in diameter. The thermometer measures the transfer of radiant energy between the surrounding surfaces and the convective heat exchange with the ambient air. The thermometer must be in place *20 minutes* before a reading can be used.

46) We selected answer A because:

The ABCs of CPR, which stands for airway, breathing and circulation, will aid you in determining what care the victim needs. Determine if the victim's airway is open. Then look, listen and feel for breathing and check for signs of circulation.

47) We selected answer C because:

Light intensity on a surface does vary inversely with the square of the distance between the source and the surface.

48) We selected answer C because:

According to 29 CFR 1910.23 A standard railing shall consist of top rail, intermediate rail, and posts, and shall have a vertical height of 42 inches nominal from upper surface of top rail to floor, platform, runway, or ramp level. The top rail shall be smooth-surfaced throughout the length of the railing. The intermediate rail shall be approximately halfway between the top rail and the floor, platform, runway, or ramp. The ends of the rails shall not overhang the terminal posts except where such overhang does not constitute a projection hazard. A standard toeboard shall be 4 inches nominal in vertical height from its top edge to the level of the floor, platform, runway, or ramp. It shall be securely fastened in place and with not more than 1/4-inch clearance above floor level. It may be made of any substantial material either solid or with openings not over 1 inch in greatest dimension.

49) We selected answer A because:

The required difference for readability is "5" feet. The use of both written text and pictographs will ensure understanding in a culturally diverse work force. Additionally, signs should be in positive terms, should be in concise easy to read terms, warn against potential hazards and signs for the same type of situation should not vary in design at the same location.

50)   We selected answer B because:

The Swinging Vane Anemometer or *Velometer* would be the instrument of choice where the exhaust opening is large and the air velocities are low as in spray booths or chemical hoods. The *rotating vane anemometer* is useful for measuring the airflow through large supply and exhaust openings where the air velocities are relatively high.

51)   We selected answer D because:

The definition of correlation is a statistical technique that measures the degree of relationship between two variables. It measures the tendency of one set of data to vary with another set of data. It does not imply a causal relationship between variables. Two sets of data that has no variation is said to have perfect correlation.

52)   We selected answer B because:

Since the company did not know about the existing problem and it was not documented, this would be treated as a new injury.

53)   We selected answer D because:

In any emergency there is a possibility that the person (or persons) involved may not be able to escape under his/her own resources. Provisions must be made for rescue by other personnel, if the need should arise. Rescues may be attempted by:

1)   Persons familiar with the product and its operation, hazards, and emergency devices.
2)   Personnel familiar with the hazards in general but not the specific equipment.
3)   Untrained personnel who are unfamiliar with the product or the hazards involved but want to help.

54)   We selected answer C because:

OSHA **1926.951(c)(1)**: Portable metal or conductive ladders shall not be used near energized lines or equipment except as may be necessary in specialized work such as in high voltage substations where nonconductive ladders might present a greater hazard than conductive ladders. Conductive or metal ladders shall be prominently marked as conductive and all necessary precautions shall be taken when used in specialized work.

55) We selected answer C because:

Hydrogen Cyanide (HCN) is a powerful asphyxiant, which would account for the red skin color. Hydrogen Cyanide also has a characteristic bitter almond smell and an IDLH of 50 ppm. Hydrogen Sulfide has a strong odor of rotten eggs. Furfural has a slight odor of almonds, as does Chlorobenzene, however they are not heavy asphyxiants.

56) We selected answer C because:

Generally, an enclosure is placed around a noise source to prevent noise from getting outside. Enclosures are normally lined with sound-absorption material to decrease internal sound pressure buildup.

57) We selected answer A because:

The cause factors discovered during accident investigations are normally corrected by the level of supervision that exercises control over the operation.

58) We selected answer C because:

Accident investigation has as its primary purpose the prevention of similar occurrences and the discovery of hazards. The intent is not to place blame or administer discipline, but rather to determine how responsibilities may be defined or clarified and to reduce error producing situations. Accident investigation should improve the safety of operations, if accident investigation is used for punitive measures, the tool has the reverse effect.

59) We selected answer B because:

1910.132(b)

Employee-owned equipment: Where employees provide their own protective equipment, the employer shall be responsible to assure its adequacy, including proper maintenance, and sanitation of such equipment.

60) We selected answer D because:

By its terms, §1926.152(a)(1) requires the use of an approved metal safety can (approved by a nationally recognized testing laboratory) for the handling and use of flammable liquids. Meeting OSHA requirements means they are either Factory Mutual (FM) approved or listed by Underwriters Laboratories, Inc. (UL), and Underwriters Laboratories Canada (ULC).Further, a safety can by definition is a container with a capacity of 5 gallons or less and equipped with a spring-closing lid and spout cover, a means to relieve internal pressure, and flash-arresting screen. According to a published memo by the OSHA Director, "we believe that DOT approved containers of 5 gallon capacity or less, although not meeting these requirements, pose very little hazard and meet the basic intent of the standard. Consequently, we have decided to exercise prosecutorial discretion and consider employer use of DOT approved containers of 5 gallon capacity or less for storage, use, and handling of flammable and combustible liquids to be de minimis noncompliance which should not be cited."

61) We selected answer A because:

This question does not include a lot of information from which to base a decision, however, we believe the best instrument would be the Combustible Gas Indicator with Oxygen sensor. This would allow the OHST to rapidly determine the presence or lack of oxygen. Obviously, one would not make an entry into an unknown area such as this without appropriate provisions for rescue and a self contained breathing apparatus.

62) We selected answer A because:

Class A fires involve ordinary combustibles. Class B fires involve flammable or combustible liquids. Class C fires involve live electrical equipment. Class D fires involve combustible metals.

Portable fire extinguishers are only designed for use on incipient fires and the employer shall provide training for all users.

63) We selected answer A because:

Although all the answers need to be addressed during the planning process, according to the NSC, "before an organization initiates an emergency plan, it should identify and evaluate the potential disasters that might occur".

64) We selected answer C because:

According to the NSC, "advanced emergency management planning is the best way to minimize potential loss from natural or human caused disasters or accidents."

65) We selected answer C because:

RCRA requires a cradle to grave system of hazardous waste management and one of the items required is the hazardous waste manifest. The hazardous waste manifest must be prepared by the generator, in sufficient copies, so that everyone handling the waste will get a copy. A final copy will be returned to the generator by the TSD who must by force of law retain a copy for three years. If after 45 days, the generator has not heard from the TSD, a notice of exception must be filed with EPA. The notice must include a copy of the manifest and an explanation of all efforts to locate the waste or manifest.

66) We selected answer B because:

EPA considers you a small quantity generator if your business produces more than 220 and less than 2,200 pounds (more than 100 and less than 1,000 kilograms) of hazardous waste in a calendar month. If you produce 1,000 kilograms or more of hazardous waste in any calendar month, or more than one kilogram of certain acutely hazardous wastes, you are subject to the more extensive regulations for large quantity generators. Large quantity generators may only store on site for a maximum of 90 days.

67) We selected answer A because:

As a link in the Chain of Custody, that is a person with a duty to preserve and protect evidence or someone with a vested interest in the outcome of the accident investigation, it is essential that from the moment the event occurs you identify, track and log movement of your evidence.

68) We selected answer D because:

1910.252(a)(2)(ii): Fire extinguishers. Suitable fire extinguishing equipment shall be maintained in a state of readiness for instant use. Such equipment may consist of pails of water, buckets of sand, hose or portable extinguishers depending upon the nature and quantity of the combustible material exposed.

69) We selected answer C because:

1910.252(b)(2)(i)(A): Helmets or hand shields shall be used during all arc welding or arc cutting operations, excluding submerged arc welding. Helpers or attendants shall be provided with proper eye protection.

1910.252(b)(2)(iii): Protection from arc welding rays. Where the work permits, the welder should be enclosed in an individual booth painted with a finish of low reflectivity such as zinc oxide (an important factor for absorbing ultraviolet radiations) and lamp black, or shall be enclosed with noncombustible screens similarly painted. Booths and screens shall permit circulation of air at floor level. Workers or other persons adjacent to the welding areas shall be protected from the rays by noncombustible or flameproof screens or shields or shall be required to wear appropriate goggles.

70) We selected answer D because:

The disorder "epicondylitis" is often called tennis elbow or sometimes carpenter's elbow. The disorder is a result of combined motion causing pronation of the hand and ulnar deviation. For a carpenter this involves swinging heavy hammers and in tennis swinging the racket. The affliction causes considerable pain in the hand, forearm and elbow. The term *rotator cuff* is associated with the tearing of a ligament in the shoulder. *Roofer's wrist* is a common name for carpal tunnel syndrome which is a disorder caused by compression of the median nerve. *Trigger finger* is an affliction caused by repeated use of the finger pulling levers or triggers, eg: paint spray operators.

71) We selected answer C because:

According to DOT regulations in 49 CFR Part 397, the shipper must:

- transport the products by truck, railroad, ship or airplane;
- determine the product's proper shipping name, hazard class, identification number, correct packaging, correct placard, and correct tables and markings;
- package the materials, label and mark the packages, prepare the shipping paper and supply the placards; and
- certify on the shipping paper that he properly complied with the rules for shipment.

72) We selected answer D because:

The activities that are required when responding to incidents can be divided into five broad interacting elements.

- **Recognition**: identification of the substance involved and the characteristics which determine the degree of hazard.
- **Evaluation**: impact or risk the substance poses to public health and the environment.
- **Control**: methods to eliminate or reduce the impact of the incident.
- **Information**: knowledge acquired concerning the conditions or circumstances particular to an incident. Information is often times

called intelligence. In a response you gather intelligence and disseminate it.

- **Safety**: protection of responders from harm.

73) We selected answer A because:

Storage using inside storage rooms must normally comply with NFPA 30 which requires that every inside storage room be equipped with one clear aisle at least three feet wide, not 22 inches as specified in answer selection "A". The standard also requires a raised 4 inch sill to prevent run off of any spilled material, self-closing fire doors and some type of exhaust system.

74) We selected answer A because:

NFPA 101, Life Safety Code, states, "A means of egress is a continuous and unobstructed way of exit travel from any point in a building or structure to a public way and consists of three separate and distinct parts: (a) the exit access, (b) the exit, and (c) the exit discharge. A means of egress comprises the vertical and horizontal travel and shall include intervening room spaces, doorways, hallways, corridors, passageways, balconies, ramps, stairs, enclosures, lobbies, escalators, horizontal exits, courts, and yards. It does not include elevators.

75) We selected answer A because:

According to 49 CFR 172.504, placards should be attached as you load and before you drive the vehicle. The placards must appear on both sides and ends of the vehicle. Each placard must be:

- easily seen from the direction it faces
- placed so the words or numbers are level and read from left to right
- at least three inches from other markings

76) We selected answer D because:

When planning for an emergency one must consider the protection of all resources. Naturally the saving of life must come first, however protection of processes and equipment is also of utmost concern. Should the decision be made to abandon hazardous processes an additional disaster could be created.

77) We selected answer B because:

According to the Life Safety Code, this is the definition of panic hardware or fire exit hardware and should be used on doors that need to be secured.

78) We selected answer A because:

Always position the command center or command post in the area of least exposure or in the cold zone.

79) We selected answer D because:

In the book *Health and Safety, Environmental and Quality Audits: A Risk-based Approach*, Though it is possible for an auditor to perform a good job within the organization with which he or she has line or staff responsibilities, it is best for an auditor to be free from all such responsibilities so that the final audit report will be perceived by all readers to be free from any real or perceived biases.

80) We selected answer A because:

A member of the management team must certify that such reviews were conducted and must include when the review was conducted and findings of applicability. This type of written certification is common practice in auditing methods because it is not practical for auditors to observe and verify that all management processes were conducted.

81) We selected answer B because:

The **Critical Incident Technique** (or **CIT**) is a set of procedures used for collecting first hand observations of human behavior that have critical significance and meet methodically defined criteria. A critical incident can be described as one that makes a significant contribution—either positively or negatively—to an activity or phenomenon and to understand the relationship between competencies and reasons for accidents. Critical incidents can be gathered in various ways, but typically respondents are asked to tell a story about an experience they have had.

Through the use of the critical incident technique one may collect specific and significant behavioral facts, providing a sound basis for making inferences as to requirements for measures of typical performance (criteria), measures of proficiency (standard samples), training, selection and classification, job design, operating procedures, equipment design, motivation and leadership (attitudes), and individual behavior. Critical incidents can be gathered in various ways, but typically respondents are asked to tell a story about an experience they have had. CIT is a flexible method that usually relies on five major areas. The first is determining and reviewing the incident, then fact-finding, which involves collecting the details of the incident from the participants. When all of the facts are collected, the next step is to identify the issues. Afterwards a decision can be made on how to resolve the issues based on various possible solutions. The final and most important aspect is the evaluation, which will determine if the solution that was selected will solve the root cause of the situation and will cause no further problems.

82) We selected Answer D because

According to Peterson's Techniques of Safety Management, only answers A, B, and C are representative of basic principles of loss control.

83) We selected Answer C because:

According to author Joe Kausek of OHSAS 18001 Designing and Implementing an Effective Health and Safety Management System, clause 4.4.4 requires electronic or hard copy of the information that provides an overall description of the main elements of the HSMS, how these elements interact and reference to any documents that describe these activities in more detail. Normally the first step in establishing control is to develop a master listing of the procedures, instructions, forms, and other documents that form the basis for the management system. This is normally called the master list. A Safety Policy Manual may serve as the Master List, but is not specifically mentioned, nor therefore required.

84)   We selected answer D because:

According to *Handbook for Professional Managers,* in the functional authority approach, the authority to act is essentially another part of whatever job is committed to take the final action or intended action. The capacity to act resides in and is part of the job. The concept of staff authority is already related to functional authority and is based solely upon the specialized knowledge and capabilities of a particular staff member (e.g., an attorney).

85)   We selected answer D because:

This standard guides how to manage and conduct quality and environmental systems, audits.

86)   We selected answer C because:

The four major elements of the U.S. OSHA Voluntary Protection Programs are (1) management commitment and employee involvement, (2) work site analysis, (3) hazard prevention and control, (4) safety and health training.

87)   We selected answer C because:

In *Essentials of Organization Behavior,* 4th Edition, managers have some discretion in the organization structural decision. Even though the strategy, size, technology, and environment constrain structural options, managers still have influence on which structure is implemented. Given this discretion and the fact that some configurations appear to influence employee performance and satisfaction, managers should consider carefully the behavioral implications when they make structural decisions.

88) We selected answer D because:

According to the *Handbook for Professional Managers,* the performance appraisal interview is more effective when the following are included:

- The supervisor indicates that the subordinate is not unusual for having a problem,
- The supervisor helps the subordinate see the importance of working on this problem,
- The supervisor helps the subordinate find a positive approach to the problem, and
- The supervisor tries to help the subordinate identify the nature of the problem, why it occurred, and its symptoms.

89) We selected answer A because:

According to the *Guidelines for Risk Based Process Safety,* A formal change analysis is essential when any kind of significant process or operational changes are anticipated. Even major equipment changes or procedural changes should induce formal and systematic change analyses. Change analysis is a form of risk assessment. Then usual formal techniques can be used (e.g., HAZOP, What-if/Checklist); however, a custom approach can also be used.

90) We selected answer B because:

The Agency of Accident is the term used in ANSI Z16.2 to identify the object, substance, or premises that contained a hazardous physical condition or circumstance.

91) We selected answer B because:

An injury is any wound or damage to the body resulting from an event in the work environment.

Examples: Cut, puncture, laceration, abrasion, fracture, bruise, contusion, chipped tooth, amputation, insect bite, electrocution, or a thermal, chemical, electrical, or radiation burn. Sprain and strain injuries to muscles, joints, and connective tissues are classified as injuries when they result from a slip, trip, fall or other similar accidents.

Pharyngitis is a respiratory condition.

92)   We selected answer D because:

Step 1:   Total the number of accidents for the period in question.

$$
\begin{array}{r}
67 \\
81 \\
98 \\
90 \\
\underline{98} \\
434
\end{array}
$$

Step 2:   Total man-hours for the same period.

$$
\begin{array}{r}
1,398,765 \\
1,456,732 \\
1,129,565 \\
1,623,451 \\
\underline{1,834,225} \\
7,442,738
\end{array}
$$

Step 3:   Apply the formula and compute the cumulative accident rate.

$$\text{Rate} = \frac{\text{H \& I Recordables} \times 200,000}{\text{Total hours worked}}$$

$$\text{Rate} = \frac{434 \times 200,000}{7,442,743}$$

$$\text{Rate} = \frac{86,800,000}{7,442,743}$$

$$\text{Rate} = 11.7$$

93) We selected answer D because:

According to the 1904.7, "Using any non-rigid means of support, such as elastic bandages, wraps, non-rigid back belts, etc. (devices with rigid stays or other systems designed to immobilize parts of the body are considered medical treatment for recordkeeping purposes) is considered first-aid.

94) We selected answer B because:

The term *incident* encompasses first-aid cases, recordable cases, restricted workday cases, lost-workday cases, permanent disability cases, near misses and property damage cases. Two basic cost categories are imperative:

Direct incident costs represent actual cash outlays attributable to the incident; such outlays would not have been necessary had the incident not occurred.

Examples of **Direct Costs** include: Workers' Compensation; Medical-Related Treatment; Medical Treatment Supplies; Ambulance Service; Drug Testing; Job Accommodations and New Equipment.

Indirect incident costs represent costs in terms of time and resources (other than cash) incurred as a result of the incident.

Examples of **Indirect Costs** include: Healthcare Professional; Injured Worker; Supervisor; Return to Work; Incident Review; Lost Production/Productivity; Human Resources; Cost to Hire; Manager; Process Delays/Interruptions; Security; Training; and Legal.

Thus, total incident costs are the sum of these individual costs.

95) We selected answer C because:

$1\% = 0.01$

0.01 times $1,000,000 = 10,000$

96) We selected answer B because:

This is a difficult question because the preferred place to conduct interviews changes with conditions. The investigator needs to make sure the witness feels at ease during the interview, which may mean conducting the interview at a location where the witness feels comfortable. However, the selected interview site must also provide privacy. Often the ideal place to interview witnesses is at the accident scene itself. This allows the witness a visual reference, fosters understanding and aids memory. Witnesses should always be interviewed individually to ensure unbiased reporting.

97) We selected answer B because:

The OSHA Asbestos Standard requires a 25 mm filter and open-face (no top) cassette and a 50 mm extension cowl on the cassette. Reference - NIOSH Analytical Method 7400.

98) We selected answer A because:

There are four major sections of the Emergency Response Guidebook that provide identification and emergency response actions. The four color-coded sections are as follows:

- The yellow-bordered section provides identification by UN/NA identification number.
- The blue-bordered section provides identification by material name.
- The orange-bordered section provides emergency response guidance.
- The green-bordered section provides initial isolation and protective action distances.

99) We selected answer C because:

Since the components are in parallel, the configuration indicates an "AND" gate situation, that is pump 1 and pump 2 must fail before hydraulic pump failure occurs. However, the calculation reveals that $(1 \times 10^{-4}) \times (1 \times 10^{-3}) = 1 \times 10^{-7}$ which is 10 times greater than the original pump failure rate. You used to have a failure once every 100 million operations, now you have a failure every 10 million operations.

100) We selected answer A because:

The mean plus two standard deviations will estimate the point at which 95.5% of the observations will fall.

Standard Deviation
Definitions

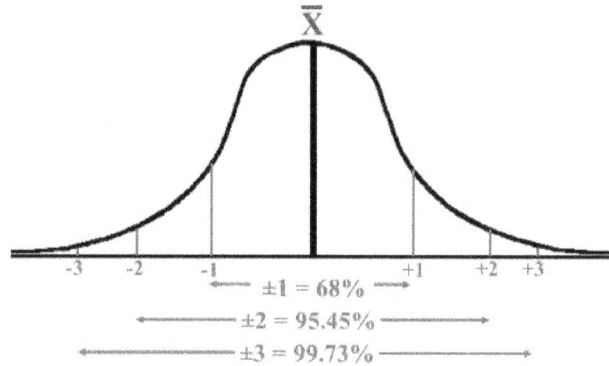

$\overline{X}$

$\pm 1 = 68\%$

$\pm 2 = 95.45\%$

$\pm 3 = 99.73\%$

-3 -2 -1 +1 +2 +3